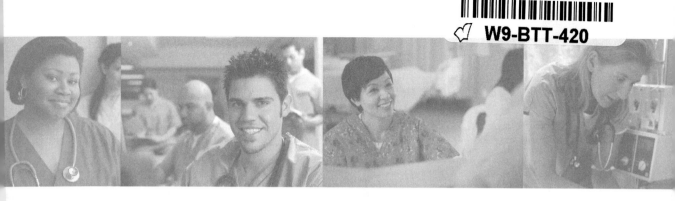

Johns Hopkins Nursing
Evidence-Based Practice:
Model and Guidelines

Second Edition

Edited by
Sandra L. Dearholt, MS, RN
Deborah Dang, PhD, RN, NEA-BC

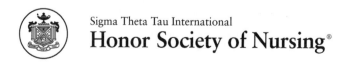

Sigma Theta Tau International
Honor Society of Nursing®

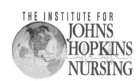

THE INSTITUTE FOR
JOHNS
HOPKINS
NURSING

Sigma Theta Tau International

The Honor Society of Nursing, Sigma Theta Tau International (STTI) is a nonprofit organization whose mission is to support the learning, knowledge, and professional development of nurses committed to making a difference in health worldwide. Founded in 1922, STTI has 130,000 members in 86 countries. Members include practicing nurses, instructors, researchers, policymakers, entrepreneurs and others. STTI's 470 chapters are located at 586 institutions of higher education throughout Australia, Botswana, Brazil, Canada, Colombia, Ghana, Hong Kong, Japan, Kenya, Malawi, Mexico, the Netherlands, Pakistan, Singapore, South Africa, South Korea, Swaziland, Sweden, Taiwan, Tanzania, the United States, and Wales. More information about STTI can be found online at www.nursingsociety.org.

Sigma Theta Tau International
550 West North Street
Indianapolis, IN, USA 46202

To order additional books, buy in bulk, or order for corporate use, contact Nursing Knowledge International at 888. NKI.4YOU (888.654.4968/US and Canada) or +1.317.634.8171 (outside US and Canada).

To request a review copy for course adoption, e-mail solutions@nursingknowledge.org or call 888.NKI.4YOU (888.654.4968/US and Canada) or +1.317.917.4983 (outside US and Canada).

To request author information, or for speaker or other media requests, contact Rachael McLaughlin of the Honor Society of Nursing, Sigma Theta Tau International at 888.634.7575 (US and Canada) or +1.317.634.8171 (outside US and Canada).

ISBN-13:   978-1-935476-59-7
EPUB and Mobi ISBN: 978-1-935476-60-3
PDF ISBN: 978-1-935476-61-0

Library of Congress Cataloging-in-Publication Data

Dearholt, Sandra.
    Johns Hopkins nursing evidence-based practice : model and guidelines / Sandra Dearholt, Deborah Dang. -- 2nd ed.
        p. ; cm.
    Nursing evidence-based practice
    Rev. ed. of: Johns Hopkins nursing evidence-based practice model and guidelines / Robin P. Newhouse ... [et al.]. c2007.
    Includes bibliographical references and index.
    ISBN 978-1-935476-76-4
    I. Dang, Deborah. II. Sigma Theta Tau International. III. Johns Hopkins University. School of Nursing. IV. Johns Hopkins nursing evidence-based practice model and guidelines. V. Title. VI. Title: Nursing evidence-based practice.
    [DNLM: 1. Evidence-Based Nursing. 2. Models, Nursing. WY 100.7]
    LC classification not assigned
    610.73--dc23
                        2011044496

Second Printing, 2012

Publisher: Renee Wilmeth
Project Editor: Billy Fields
Copy Editor: Kevin Kent
Indexer: Johnna Dinse
Second Edition Cover Design: Katy Bodenmiller
Original Cover Designer: Studio Galou

Principal Book Editor: Carla Hall
Editorial Coordinator: Paula Jeffers
Proofreader: Barbara Bennett
Interior Design: Rebecca Batchelor
Page Layout: Rebecca Batchelor

Praise for *Johns Hopkins Nursing Evidence-Based Practice Model and Guidelines, Second Edition*

"*Johns Hopkins Nursing Evidence-Based Practice Model and Guidelines*, Second Edition, provides an outstanding foundation for practice based on using evidence to guide decision-making. Clinical nurses with diverse educational preparation can successfully use this process and incorporate evidence-based changes into their practice. Strategies are provided on how to create and build a supportive environment and culture in which EBP can thrive."

–LeeAnna Spiva, PhD, RN, PLNC
Director of Nursing Research
WellStar Development Center, Center for Nursing Excellence

"The Johns Hopkins Nursing Evidence-Based Practice model exemplifies the values driving today's health care world. PET provides a step-by-step process for incorporating evidence into practice and recognizes the importance of an interdisciplinary team in improving patient care. This book offers a comprehensive guide to using evidence to improve practice, with real examples of successful translation that are applicable to all levels of nursing."

–Nancy Wells, DNSc, RN, FAAN
Director of Nursing Research
Vanderbilt University Medical Center
Nashville, Tennessee

–Victoria Sandlin, MSN, RN
Research Nurse III, Nursing Research Program
Vanderbilt University Medical Center
Nashville, Tennessee

"*Johns Hopkins Nursing Evidence-Based Practice Model and Guidelines*, Second Edition, takes the fear out of EBP and demonstrates for the nurse how simple it can be. The three-step 'PET' process simplifies it so that a nurse can break the steps down, instead of feeling overwhelmed by the entire process."

–Debra Sheets, MN, RN, NEA-BC
Director, Special Projects
Peninsula Regional Medical Center

"The Johns Hopkins Nursing Evidence-Based Practice model provides a practical, step-by-step framework that will help elevate nursing practice at all levels from 'what we have always done' to evidence-based patient care. This important book provides the relevant tools and clinical examples to support this cultural transition to improved patient outcomes and will help build nurse leaders in the process."

–Jenny Richardson, MS, RN, CNS
Clinical Nurse Specialist, Primary Care Division
Portland Veterans Affairs Medical Center

"The authors of this second edition provide even further depth and clarification to the Johns Hopkins Nursing Evidence-Based Practice model, which our health system has adopted. The advancements in appraisal methods and translation pathways empower nurses at all levels to participate in the vital work of EBP, from the bedside to the boardroom."

–Miki Goodwin, PhD, RN, PHN
Director, Center for Nursing Evidence-Based Practice,
Research, and Innovation
St. Luke's Health System, Treasure Valley
Boise, Idaho

"We have greatly benefitted from using the practical, user-friendly approach to EBP that the first edition of this book provided, which led to our own adoption of the JHNEBP model for nursing practice. The new edition provides even more nuggets of wisdom, experience, practical how-tos, and examples that will help the clinical nurse learn how to apply current best evidence to his or her practice. The appendices now include more detailed explanations of how to use each tool. This book is a must-read for all health care practitioners, leaders, and students who wish to effectively move through the continuum of practice question to translation."

–Walter Lewanowicz, MN, RN
Nurse Educator, VCU Health System
Adjunct Faculty, VCU School of Nursing

DEDICATION

This book is dedicated to those nurses everywhere—consummate professionals in whatever setting they practice—who are committed to excellence in patient care based on the best available evidence.

ACKNOWLEDGEMENTS

We would like to acknowledge the insight and expertise of the authors of the first edition (2007) of *Johns Hopkins Nursing Evidence-Based Practice Model and Guidelines*: **Robin P. Newhouse**, PhD, RN, NEA-BC, FAAN; **Sandra L. Dearholt**, MS, RN; **Stephanie S. Poe**, DNP, RN; **Linda C. Pugh**, PhD, RNC, CNE, FAAN; and **Kathleen M. White**, PhD, RN, NEA-BC, FAAN.

The foundational work of these experts transformed evidence-based practice into a process that promotes autonomy and provides bedside nurses with the competencies and tools to apply the best evidence to improve patient care. The profession as a whole is indebted to them.

ABOUT THE EDITORS

Sandra L. Dearholt

Sandra L. Dearholt, MS, RN, is Assistant Director of Nursing for the Departments of Neurosciences and Psychiatry Nursing at The Johns Hopkins Hospital. Ms. Dearholt has written a variety of articles on evidence-based practice (EBP) and has extensive experience in the development and delivery of EBP educational programs. Her areas of interest focus on strategies for incorporating EBP into practice at the bedside, the development of professional practice standards, and fostering service excellence. She is a co-author of the first edition of *Johns Hopkins Nursing Evidence-Based Practice: Model and Guidelines* and a contributing author to *Johns Hopkins Nursing Evidence-Based Practice: Implementation and Translation.*

Deborah Dang

Deborah Dang, PhD, RN, NEA-BC, is Director of Nursing Practice, Education, and Research at The Johns Hopkins Hospital. She developed the strategic vision for EBP at The Johns Hopkins Hospital and built an infrastructure that enabled the transformation to practice based on evidence. Dr. Dang has published, consulted, and presented nationally and internationally on the subject of EBP. She is a contributing author to *Johns Hopkins Nursing Evidence-Based Practice: Implementation and Translation.* She also holds a Joint Appointment with The Johns Hopkins University School of Nursing. As a health services researcher, her funded studies focus on disruptive clinician behavior in hospitals, and leadership performance based on a framework of positive psychology.

ABOUT THE CONTRIBUTING AUTHORS

Chapter 1: Evidence-Based Practice: Context, Concerns, and Challenges

Linda C. Pugh, PhD, RNC, FAAN

Linda Pugh is a Professor of Nursing at the York College of Pennsylvania, the Director of the Graduate Programs in Nursing, and the past Director of Evidence-based Practice/Nursing Research at the York Hospital. Dr. Pugh co-authored the first edition of *Johns Hopkins Nursing Evidence-Based Practice: Model and Guidelines*. As a certified obstetric nurse, she has provided care for childbearing women for over 30 years. She has been the recipient of numerous grants to support her research on improving breastfeeding outcomes particularly with low-income women. She has published and presented her work nationally and internationally.

Chapter 2: Critical Thinking and Evidence-Based Practice

Anne E. Belcher, PhD, RN, AOCN, ANEF, FAAN

Anne Belcher is Associate Professor and Director, Office for Teaching Excellence, at The Johns Hopkins University School of Nursing. She has more than 40 years of experience in nursing education, having taught at the baccalaureate, master's and doctoral levels. She has held numerous administrative and educator positions throughout her career, receiving the National League for Nursing Excellence in Teaching Award in 2009. Dr. Belcher's area of expertise is oncology nursing, and her research interest is psychosocial aspects of cancer, with a focus on spiritual care.

Zeina E. Khouri-Stevens, PhD, RN

Zeina Khouri-Stevens is the Director of Nursing for inpatient surgery and neurosciences for The Johns Hopkins Bayview Medical Center. Dr. Khouri has published on such topics as shared decision-making and patient safety. Her research interests include the relationship between critical thinking and critical decision-making and mindfulness.

Chapter 3: The Johns Hopkins Nursing Evidence-Based Practice Model and Process Overview

Sandra L. Dearholt, MS, RN

> See Sandra L. Dearholt's bio on page vi.

Chapter 4: The Practice Question

Robin P. Newhouse, PhD, RN, NEA-BC, FAAN

> Robin Newhouse is Associate Professor and Chair, Organizational Systems and Adult Health at the University of Maryland School of Nursing. She has published, presented, and consulted nationally and internationally on the topic of evidence-based nursing practice. Dr. Newhouse co-authored the first edition of *The Johns Hopkins Nursing Evidence-Based Practice: Model and Guidelines*. As a health services researcher, her funded studies focus on the translation of evidence to practice and the effect of nursing care on patient outcomes. Dr. Newhouse is a member of the American Nurses Credentialing Center's Research Council and is past Chair of the Research and Scholarship Advisory Council for Sigma Theta Tau International, the Honor Society of Nursing.

Stephanie S. Poe, DNP, RN

> Stephanie Poe is the Director of Nursing Clinical Quality and Chief Nursing Information Officer at the Johns Hopkins Hospital. Dr. Poe co-authored the first edition of the *Johns Hopkins Nursing Evidence-Based Practice: Model and Guidelines* and co-edited *Johns Hopkins Nursing Evidence-Based Practice: Implementation and Translation*.

Chapter 5: Searching for Evidence

Emily Munchel, RN, CPN

> Emily Munchel is a Nurse Clinician at The Johns Hopkins Hospital and led the implementation of EBP on an inpatient pediatric unit in The Johns Hopkins Hospital Children's Center. She was an EBP Fellow and in that role mentored, taught, and led EBP projects for clinical nursing departments at The Johns Hopkins Hospital.

Stella Seal, MLS

Stella Seal is Operations Manager for the William H. Welch Medical Library, The Johns Hopkins University. She has served as a liaison to the School of Nursing and Nursing Administration since 2002. She is an expert in searching databases for biomedical literature, and serves as both an educator and consultant for literature searches that support research, education, and patient care goals.

Christina L. Wissinger, MS, MLIS

Christina Wissinger has worked in academic health sciences libraries for over four years and has collaborated with the nursing community at The Johns Hopkins University in addition to allied health professionals, clinicians, and biomedical researchers as part of her work. Ms. Wissinger has conducted numerous training sessions on a wide variety of research tools, collaborated on grant-funded research and non-funded systematic reviews and has created several training sessions for continuing education credits in the areas of pharmacy and physical medicine and rehabilitation.

Chapter 6: Evidence Appraisal: Research

Stephanie S. Poe, DNP, RN

See Stephanie S. Poe's bio on page viii.

Linda Costa, PhD, RN, NEA-BC

Linda Costa is Nurse Researcher at The Johns Hopkins Hospital, Assistant Professor at The JHU School of Nursing, and a member of The Johns Hopkins Medicine Institutional Review Board. Dr. Costa has presented widely on the topics of evidence-based practice and research. She is a contributing author to *Johns Hopkins Nursing Evidence-Based Practice: Implemntation and Translation.* Her program of research is focused on self-management of complex medication regimens during care transitions.

Chapter 7: Evidence Appraisal: Non-Research

Sarah J. M. (Jodi) Shaefer, PhD, RN

Sarah Shaefer is an Assistant Professor, Department of Community-Public Health at The Johns Hopkins University School of Nursing and Nurse Researcher, The Johns Hopkins Bayview Medical Center. Dr. Shaefer significantly expanded collaboration between bedside and student nurses on EBP projects and has presented student satisfaction data with these collaborations internationally.

Hayley D. Mark, PhD, MPH, RN

Hayley D. Mark is an Assistant Professor at The Johns Hopkins University School of Nursing and a member of the Johns Hopkins Medicine Institutional Review Board. She has taught research methods to nursing students for over six years. Dr. Mark's research focus is in sexually transmitted disease and behavior change. She has also presented on the topics of evidence-based practice and research and published and presented her work nationally and internationally.

Chapter 8: Translation

Robin P. Newhouse, PhD, RN, NEA-BC, FAAN

See Robin P. Newhouse's bio on page viii.

Kathleen White, PhD, RN, NEA-BC, FAAN

Kathleen White is an Associate Professor at The Johns Hopkins University School of Nursing. Dr. White has authored multiple publications on the Johns Hopkins Nursing EBP model and also consults and presents on this subject. Dr. White co-authored the first edition of *Johns Hopkins Nursing Evidence-Based Practice: Model and Guidelines* and co-edited *Johns Hopkins Nursing Evidence-Based Practice: Implementation and Translation*.

Chapter 9: Creating a Supportive EBP Environment

Kathleen White, PhD, RN, NEA-BC, FAAN

> See Kathleen White's bio on page x.

Deborah Dang, PhD, RN, NEA-BC

> See Deborah Dang's bio on page vi.

Chapter 10: Exemplars

Maria Cvach, MS, RN, CCRN

> Maria Cvach is the Assistant Director of Nursing for Clinical Standards at The Johns Hopkins Hospital and the chair of the EBP Steering Committee for Johns Hopkins Hospital. She has extensive experience facilitating EBP projects, and authored a chapter in *Johns Hopkins Nursing Evidence-Based Practice: Implementation and Translation.* In addition, Maria has 17 years of experience as a Nurse Educator and has presented nationally on various topics, including critical care, alarm management, fall prevention, and EBP.

Support Surfaces and Pressure Ulcers

> Rachel N. Moseley, RN, CWON, CWCN
> Wound Ostomy Nurse Specialist
> Johns Hopkins Bayview Medical Center
> Baltimore, MD, USA
>
> Cynthia A. Walker, RN, CWON
> Wound Ostomy Nurse Specialist
> Johns Hopkins Bayview Medical Center
> Baltimore, MD, USA
>
> Mary Ann Greene, DNP, RN, NEA-BC
> Director of Education and Practice
> Johns Hopkins Bayview Medical Center
> Baltimore, MD, USA

Zeina Khouri-Stevens, PhD, RN
Johns Hopkins Bayview Medical Center
Baltimore, MD, USA

Maria Koszalka, EdD, RN
Vice President, Patient Care Services
Johns Hopkins Bayview Medical Center
Baltimore, MD, USA

Sarah J. M. Shaefer, PhD, RN

Use of Evidence-Based Practice Model by a Professional Nursing Association

Paula Graling, DrNP, CNS, RN, CNOR
Chair of the Evidence Rating Task Force – AORN
Association of periOperative Registered Nurses
Denver, CO, USA

Placing Patients Taking Oral Anti-Platelet Medications on Bleeding Precautions

Maria Cvach, MS, RN, CCRN
Emily Munchel, RN, CPN

Fall Injury Risk Assessment

Maria Cvach, MS, RN, CCRN

Patricia B. Dawson, MSN, RN
Assistant Director, Nursing Clinical Quality and Magnet
The Johns Hopkins Hospital
Baltimore, MD, USA

Preventing Pediatric Infiltrates

Lori D. Van Gosen, MSN, RN, CRNI
Nurse Clinician III
The Johns Hopkins Hospital
Baltimore, MD, USA

The Frequency of Manufactured Intravenous Fluid Bag Replacement

Emily Munchel, RN, CPN

Regina Hendrix, MSN, MPA, RN-BC
Coordinator of Nursing Education, Medical Nursing
The Johns Hopkins Hospital
Baltimore, MD, USA

Keisha Perrin, RN
Nurse Clinician III
The Johns Hopkins Hospital
Baltimore, MD, USA

Shilta Subhas, MS, RN
Clinical Nurse Specialist
The Johns Hopkins Hospital
Baltimore, MD, USA

Kathy Wagner-Kosmakos, MS, RN
Assistant Director, Regulatory Affairs
Patient Care Services
The Johns Hopkins Hospital
Baltimore, MD, USA

Ankyloglossia, Frenotomy and Breast Feeding

Deborah Dixon, RN, IBCLC
Lactation Consultant Coordinator
The Johns Hopkins Hospital
Baltimore, MD, USA

Kathleen White, PhD, RN, NEA-BC, FAAN

TABLE OF CONTENTS

Appendixes

FOREWORD

Nursing has long been described as both an art and a science: an art grounded in personal commitment, long-standing tradition, and clinical expertise and a science encompassing a distinct body of knowledge, practice disciplines, goals, and methodologies. The distinction is in the details.

Nursing as an art, heavily dependent on an individual's skills and abilities, is creative and compassionate at its best. It can, however, become prey to provincial thinking. "I've always done it this way" can be an unhealthy mindset in a rapidly expanding and complex field. Evidence-based practice supports the science of nursing, providing high-quality patient care based on the best available evidence. Using a formal process, nurses access, synthesize, and translate the research and thinking of a wide range of experts and disciplines into their practice.

This second edition of *Johns Hopkins Nursing Evidence-Based Practice: Model and Guidelines* must echo the Foreword from the first:

> *"Evidence-based practice is important to the safety of our patients, the development of our profession, and the education of our students."*

It is a tribute to the 2007 edition, created and tested by a team of nurses and faculty at The Johns Hopkins Hospital and The Johns Hopkins University School of Nursing, that this second edition was conceived. Hundreds of health care professionals have used the model in a variety of settings, from hospitals and schools of nursing to professional organizations both in and outside the nursing arena. These dedicated practitioners have used the model, consulted with the authors and other practitioners, shared insights in appraising evidence, and reflected on their experience of applying the model in clinical settings. Their feedback, in turn, has enhanced our understanding of the model and contributed to a revision of the tools in this edition.

The model and guidelines provide a process for formulating a practice question, appraising research and non-research evidence, and making recommendations for practice. The recommendations direct a course of action incorporating the best evidence into patient care.

We are proud to endorse this second edition of *Johns Hopkins Nursing Evidence-Based Practice: Model and Guidelines*. We hope it will enhance both the art and the science of your nursing care.

Karen Haller, PhD, RN, FAAN
Vice President for Nursing and Patient Care Services,
Chief Nursing Officer
The Johns Hopkins Hospital
Baltimore, Maryland, USA

Martha N. Hill, PhD, RN, FAAN
Dean, The Johns Hopkins University School of Nursing
Baltimore, Maryland, USA

Introduction

The Johns Hopkins Nursing Evidence-Based Practice: Model and Guidelines is dedicated to the advancement of evidence-based practice (EBP). The second edition was written to reflect advancements in the appraisal and synthesis of evidence over the past five years. In today's complex and dynamic patient care environment, the need for nursing interventions and processes informed by the best evidence remains vital to realizing health care improvements and cost savings. Our intent, as with the first edition, is to present a guided approach to evidence-based practice for the bedside clinician. Whereas the first edition was based on our experience at The Johns Hopkins Hospital and The Johns Hopkins University School of Nursing, this edition reflects our learning from bedside nurses and students that we interacted with over the years.

Part I introduces the EBP concept, including its evolution within the nursing profession, and recasts the context to reflect demands for nursing practice based on evidence and the challenges presented by changes, such as 1) health care reform and 2) the Institute of Medicine's *The Future of Nursing: Leading Change, Advancing Health Care* report recommendation that nurses fully partner with physicians and other health care professionals in redesigning health care in the United States.

Part II includes an updated overview of the Johns Hopkins Nursing Evidence-based Practice Model and process and reflects how EBP has been incorporated into national nursing standards and links to nursing excellence through Magnet recognition.

Part III expands the description of the importance of the problem statement and the PICO format. It enhances the content of appraising research and non-research evidence, assessing the quality of evidence and the synthesis process. Content related to the use of translation pathways has been included to guide decision-making for practice changes.

Part IV discusses how to select an EBP model and explores how to create and build a supportive environment in which EBP can flourish. It describes strategies for establishing a culture of practice based on evidence, developing staff and organizational capacity and sustainability.

Part V provides new exemplars of hospital-based EBP projects and includes application of the model within a professional nursing organization.

Part VI contains redesigned tools and guides that assist clinicians in applying the EBP process. The tools and guides include directions for use and comprehensive criteria for identifying the strength and quality of the evidence.

With the second edition, we hope to spread the knowledge and experience gained by the many nurses who used *The Johns Hopkins Nursing Evidence-Based Practice: Model and Guidelines* to enhance their practice for the benefit of their patients. This work carries on a tradition voiced by M. Adelaide Nutting, Johns Hopkins nurse and pioneer in the development of nursing education:

> *We need to realize and affirm a view that "medicine" is one of the most difficult of arts. Compassion may provide the motive but knowledge is our only working power.... Surely we will not be satisfied with merely perpetuating methods and traditions; surely we should be more and more involved in creating them.*

Evidence-Based Practice
Background

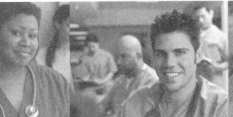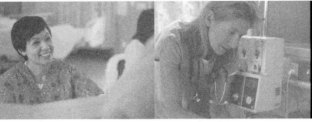

Evidence-Based Practice: Context, Concerns, and Challenges

Linda C. Pugh, PhD, RNC, FAAN

Evidence-based practice (EBP) positions nurses to have a significant influence on health care decisions and become partners in improving quality of care. Beyond an expectation for professional practice, EBP provides a major opportunity for nurses to enlighten practice and add value to the patient experience. The Institute of Medicine (IOM, 2003) published a report about the education of health professionals highlighting five core competencies: patient-centered care, quality improvement, informatics, *evidence-based practice,* and work in interprofessional teams. The Institute (IOM, 2010) also advocated that nurses become full partners in the redesign of health care systems to improve the quality of practice. This report suggests nurses need a strong foundation in *evidence-based* care to accomplish this goal. Further, Dr. Patricia A. Grady, Director of the National Institute for Nursing Research, stated that "nurse scientists are well positioned to take leadership roles and serve as catalysts" in the field of translational science, that is, translating research into everyday practice (Grady, 2010, p. 166). Perhaps the strongest support for addressing a health care system dedicated to providing the best care with the best outcomes was proposed by the *Quality and Safety Education for Nurses* (QSEN) project funded by the Robert Wood Johnson Foundation. The QSEN project has identified core competencies for *all* registered nurses (Cronenwett, et al., 2007). These competencies are patient-centered care, teamwork and collaboration, *evidence-based practice*, quality improvement, safety, and informatics. Using the best evidence to provide health care is critical to realizing health care improvements and cost savings. The objectives for this chapter are to

- Define evidence-based practice
- Describe the evolution of EBP in the nursing profession
- Discuss EBP in relation to outcomes, accountability, and translation to practice
- Highlight nursing's role in evidence-based practice

EBP: A Definition

EBP is a problem-solving approach to clinical decision-making within a health care organization. It integrates the best available scientific evidence with the best available experiential (patient and practitioner) evidence. EBP considers internal and external influences on practice and encourages critical thinking in the judicious application of such evidence to the care of individual patients, a patient population, or a system (Newhouse, Dearholt, Poe, Pugh, & White, 2007). The challenge for health care providers is to use research and non-research evidence to implement the best interventions and practices.

EBP supports and informs clinical, administrative, and educational decision-making. Combining research, organizational experience (including quality improvement, program and evaluation data), clinical expertise, expert opinion, and patient preferences ensures clinical decisions based on all available evidence. EBP enhances *efficacy* (the ability to reach a desired result); *efficiency* (the achievement of a desired result with minimum expense, time, and effort); and *effectiveness* (the ability to produce a desired result). Additionally, EBP weighs risk, benefit, and cost against a backdrop of patient preferences. This decision-making encourages health care providers to question practice and determine which interventions work and which do not. EBP ensures health care providers use evidence to promote optimal outcomes or equivalent care at lower cost or in less time and to promote patient satisfaction and higher health-related quality of life.

Differentiating Quality Improvement, Research, and EBP

Nurses are often perplexed about differences between quality improvement, EBP, and research. Quality improvement (QI) is a process by which individuals work to improve systems and processes at the local level (i.e., unit, department, organization) with the intent to improve outcomes (Committee on Assessing the System for Protecting Human Research Participants, 2002). QI generally includes a method of measuring a particular outcome, making changes to improve practice, and monitoring performance on an ongoing basis. QI may uncover a practice problem that initiates an EBP project. Some examples of QI initiatives include decreasing falls among patients, decreasing surgical-site infections, improving patient satisfaction, improving pneumococcal and influenza immunization rates, and decreasing restraint use.

Research is a systematic investigation designed to generate or contribute to new knowledge that can be generalized for broader application (Department of Health and Human Services, 2005, 45 CFR 46.102[d]). It is often undertaken when no evidence is found during an EBP project. Some examples of research include investigating pain in the ventilated patient; communication between caregivers, family, and patient at the end of life; and post-stroke memory function.

An EBP project is often undertaken when QI indicates a practice problem or when clinicians have a particular concern or question about their practice. The EBP process includes recruiting an interprofessional team to develop and refine the EBP question, applying a rigorous search strategy to locate best available evidence, appraising the strength and quality of evidence, and synthesizing findings leading to evidence-based practice recommendations. Some examples include performing mouth care every four hours on ventilated patients because the literature shows it helps decrease incidence of ventilator-associated pneumonia and decreases mortality, cost, and length of stay and using warm water compresses to manage nipple pain in breastfeeding mothers.

The History

EBP is not conceptually new; its roots extend back many decades. However, as with any applied science, the terms associated with evidence-based practice changed as the science evolved. As early as 1972, Archibald L. Cochrane, a British epidemiologist, criticized the health profession for administering treatments not supported by evidence (Cochrane, 1972). By the 1980s, the term *evidence-based medicine* was being used at McMaster University Medical School in Canada. Positive reception given to systematic reviews of care during pregnancy and childbirth prompted the British National Health Service in 1992 to approve funding for "a Cochrane Centre" to facilitate the preparation of systematic reviews of randomized controlled trials of health care, eventually leading to the establishment of the Cochrane Collaboration in 1993 (The Cochrane Collaboration, 2011). The Cochrane Collaboration provides systematic reviews about the effectiveness of health care. These reviews provide logical reasoning and sound evidence for providing effective treatment regimes.

Building on these early efforts, evidence-based practice has developed to include increasingly sophisticated analytical techniques; improved presentation and dissemination of information; growing knowledge of how to implement findings while effectively considering patient preferences, costs, and policy issues; and better understanding of how to measure effect and use feedback to promote ongoing improvement.

Research Utilization

More than 30 years ago, the Western Interstate Commission for Higher Education (WICHE) initiated the first major nurse-based EBP project (Krueger, 1978) to use research in the clinical setting. Research, a relatively new professional discipline for nurses, was just beginning to develop; nurses were interested in conducting research useful to clinicians. The outcomes of the 6-year WICHE project were not as favorable as had been anticipated. Nursing science targeted the study of nurses at the time, and finding interventions to use in practice was difficult.

The Conduct and Utilization of Research in Nursing Project (CURN) began in the 1970s (Horsley, Crane, & Bingle, 1978). Ten areas were identified as having adequate evidence to use in practice (CURN Project, 1981–1982):

- Structured preoperative teaching
- Reducing diarrhea in tube-fed patients
- Preoperative sensory preparation to promote recovery
- Prevention of decubitus ulcers
- Intravenous cannula change
- Closed urinary drainage systems
- Distress reduction through sensory preparation
- Mutual goal setting in patient care
- Clean intermittent catheterization
- Pain: Deliberate nursing interventions

The actual translation of research into practice has been slowly taking place since the 1960s. In 2006, National Institute for Nursing Research (NINR) published 10 landmark programs that have had a major impact on health care (www. nih/ninr.gov/). (See Table 1.1.)

Table 1.1   NINR Nursing Research Programs That Impacted Health Care

Nurse Scientist	Topic	Findings
Dr. Linda Aiken, 2002	Nurse staffing	Lower patient mortality is linked to higher nurse staffing levels. Appropriate numbers of nurses improves patient safety.

Table 1.1   NINR Nursing Research Programs That Impacted Health Care (continued)

Nurse Scientist	Topic	Findings
Dr. Nancy Bergstrom, 1996	Pressure sores	Identifying patients at risk for pressure sores using a reliable and valid instrument (Braden Scale) prevents pressure sores. Such identification, therefore, results in fewer debilitating pressure sores, saves money, and improves the patient's quality of life.
Dr. Margaret Grey, 2001	Teens who cope with diabetes	Providing coping skills training for teenagers with diabetes leads to better control and improvement in long-term blood sugar levels. Managing chronic illness leads to better outcomes for these adolescents.
Dr. Joanne S. Harrell, 1996	Lifestyle behaviors (exercise and diet) for children and youth	Programs to enhance cardiovascular health among children and youth are strategies that can lower cholesterol and body fat. Increasing physical activity among the nation's youth may decrease early development of cardiovascular disease.
Dr. Martha N. Hill, 2003	Reducing the risk of hypertension among young urban black men	A team of health care workers provided access to hypertensive medications, follow-up care, home visits, and referrals. Participants had lower systolic and diastolic blood pressures and fewer signs of heart or kidney damage. A trusting relationship resulted in lifestyle changes which ultimately improved health.

Table 1.1   NINR Nursing Research Programs That Impacted Health Care (continued)

Nurse Scientist	Topic	Findings
Dr. Loretta Sweet Jemmott, 1998	Reducing the risk of HIV among young minority women	Educational interventions are effective in decreasing risky behaviors. This program has been translated both nationally and internationally as a model curriculum.
Drs. Jon Levine and Christine Miaskowski, 1999	Pain responses and the management of pain	Gender may influence pain response and should be considered in developing effective strategies to manage pain.
Dr. Kate Lorig, 1999	Managing chronic illness (such as arthritis) among older Hispanics	A self-management program demonstrated increased understanding of chronic disease and increased activity levels among participants, resulting in an improvement in their quality of life.
Dr. Mary D. Naylor, 2004	Improving the outcomes for the elderly after hospital discharge	The transitional care model improved the health of elders and was demonstrated to be cost effective.
Dr. David Olds, 1997	Home nurse visitation improves health outcomes of low-income mothers and children	Low-income women who were visited by nurses frequently during their pregnancies had improved health outcomes. Their children also had multiple benefits, such as higher IQ scores and fewer behavioral problems.

EBP and Outcomes

Health care providers, by nature, have always been interested in the outcomes and results of patient care. Traditionally, such results have been characterized in terms of morbidity and mortality. Recently, however, the focus has broadened to include *clinical outcomes* (e.g., treatments), *functional outcomes* (e.g., performance of daily activities), *quality of life outcomes* (e.g., patient satisfaction), and *economic outcomes* (e.g., direct, indirect, and intangible costs). EBP is an explicit process by which clinicians conduct critical evidence reviews and examine the link between health care practices and outcomes to inform decisions and improve quality of care.

EBP and Accountability

Nowhere is accountability a more sensitive topic than in health care. Knowing that patient outcomes are linked to evidence-based interventions is critical for promoting quality patient care, is mandated by professional and regulatory organizations and third-party payers, and is expected by patients and families.

Much of the information available suggests consumers are not consistently receiving appropriate care (IOM, 2001). Public expectations that health care investments lead to high-quality results most likely will not diminish in the near future. Because quality and cost concerns drive health care, nurses, like other professionals, must operate within an age of accountability (McQueen & Mc-Cormick, 2001); this accountability has become a focal point for health care (Pronovost, 2010). It is within this environment that nurses, physicians, public health scientists, and others explore what works and does not, and it is within this context that nurses and other health care providers continue the journey to bridge research and practice.

Governments and society challenge health care providers to base their practices on current, validated interventions (Zerhouni, 2006). In 2011, the Director of the National Institutes of Health, Dr. Francis S. Collins, proposed the National Center for Advancing Translational Sciences. Dr. Collins addressed the importance of moving basic bench research into everyday practice (Collins, 2011). EBP is one response to this mandate and a logical progression in the continuing effort to close the gap between research and practice (Grady, 2010; Titler, 2004; Weaver, Warren, & Delaney, 2005).

Nurses are accountable for the interventions they provide, and EBP provides a systematic approach to decision-making that leads to best practices and demonstrates such accountability. When the strongest available evidence is considered, the odds of doing the right thing at the right time for the right patient are improved. Given the complexity of linking research and clinical practice, the definitions and concepts associated with EBP have developed over time and can vary according to the theoretical framework adopted. Still, EBP provides the most useful framework born of collaborative efforts to translate evidence into practice.

Translation of Evidence

Translation involves the synthesis, implementation, evaluation, and dissemination of research and non-research evidence. EBP has evolved through the measurement of outcomes and the analysis of the overall conditions that foster individual patient and system-wide improvements. Nurses need to evaluate whether or not evidence from translation efforts provides insights that contribute to patient care. Such an evaluation would also determine whether or not best practice information (such as clinical practice guidelines) is useful when addressing complex clinical questions within their specific health care setting. Measuring improvements and determining the most appropriate way to affect policy is necessary. EBP depends on the collective capacity of nurses to develop cultures of critical thinking where ongoing learning is inherent. As the field evolves, nurses can serve patients and the profession by exploring translation processes and promoting the use of evidence in routine decisions to improve practice outcomes.

Knowing and Using Evidence

In health care, unfortunately, more is known than is practiced. The process of incorporating new knowledge into clinical practice is often considerably delayed. Collins (2011) reports that it takes on average 13 years to approve new drugs. Balus and Boren (2000) suggests it can take up to 17 years before new research findings become part of clinical practice.

New knowledge has grown exponentially. Early in the 20th century, professional nurses had but a few, hard to access journals available to them. Today,

MEDLINE indexes 5,484 journals (National Library of Medicine, 2011) with over 21 million citations. The Cumulative Index to Nursing and Allied Health Literature (CINAHL) indexes 4,600 journals (Ebsco Publishing, 2011). Accessibility of information on the Web also has increased consumer expectation of participating in treatment decisions. Patients with chronic health problems have accumulated considerable expertise in self-management, increasing the pressure for providers to be up-to-date with the best evidence for care.

Despite this knowledge explosion, health care clinicians can experience a decline in knowledge of best care practices that relates to the amount of information available and the limited time to digest it. Studies show knowledge of best care practices negatively correlates with year of graduation—that is, knowledge of best care practices declines as the number of years since the nurse's graduation increases (Estabrooks, 1998; Shin, Haynes, & Johnston, 1993). EBP is one of the best strategies to enable nurses to stay abreast of new practices and technology amidst this continuing information explosion.

Nursing's Role in EBP

EBP encompasses multiple sources of knowledge, clinical expertise, and patient preference. Because of their unique position and expertise at the bedside, nurses often play a pivotal role in generating questions about patient care and safety. This, along with the fact that practice questions and concerns often cross disciplines, makes it critical to enlist an interprofessional team and to include patient and family input as part of the process. Thus, nurses need to develop the necessary knowledge and skills not only to participate in an EBP process, but to serve as leaders of interdisciplinary EBP teams seeking best practices to improve patient care. Nurses and nursing leaders also play a central role in modeling and promoting a culture that supports the use of collaborative EBP within the organization and in ensuring that the necessary resources (e.g., time, education, equipment, mentors, and library support) are in place to facilitate and sustain the process.

Summary

This chapter defines EBP and discusses the evolution that led to the critical need for practice based on evidence to guide decision-making. EBP creates a culture of critical thinking and ongoing learning and is the foundation for an environment where evidence supports clinical, administrative, and educational decisions. EBP supports rational decision-making, reducing inappropriate variation and making it easier for nurses to do their job.

Numbering more than 3 million and practicing in all health care settings, nurses make up the largest number of health professionals. Every patient is likely to receive nursing care; therefore, nurses are in a position to influence the type, quality, and cost of care provided to patients. For nursing, the framework for decision-making has traditionally been the nursing process. Understood in this framework is the use of evidence to guide the nurse in the planning for and making decisions about care. EBP is an explicit process that facilitates meeting the needs of patients and delivering care that is effective, efficient, equitable, patient-centered, safe, and timely (IOM, 2001).

References

Balas, E.A. & Boren, S.A. (2000) Managing clinical knowledge for healthcare improvement. In J. Bemmel & A.T. McCray (Eds.) yearbook of Medical Informatics (pp. 65-70). Bethesda, MD: National Library of Medicine.

Cochrane, A. L. (1972). *Effectiveness and efficiency: Random reflections on health services.* London: Nuffield Provincial Hospitals Trust. The Cochrane Collaboration.

The Cochrane Collaboration. (2011). Retrieved from http://www.cochrane.org/about-us/history

Collins, F. S. (2011). Reengineering translational science: The time is right. *Science Translational Medicine,* 3(90), 90cm17.

Committee on Assessing the System for Protecting Human Research Participants. (2002). *Responsible research: A systems approach to protecting research participants.* Washington, DC: The National Academies Press.

Cronenwett, L., Sherwood, G., Barnsteiner, J., Disch, J., Johnson, J., Mitchell, P., Sullivan, D. T., & Warren, J. (2007). Quality and safety education for nurses. *Nursing Outlook,* 55(3), 122-131. Doi: 10.1016/j.outlook.2007.02.006.

Department of Health and Human Services. (2005). Code of Federal Regulations Title 45 Public Welfare Part 46 Protection of Human Subjects. Retrieved from http://www.hhs.gov/ohrp/policy/ohrpregulations.pdf

Ebsco Publishing. (2011). CINAHL Plus Full Text. Retrieved from http://www.ebscohost.com/academic/cinahl-plus-with-full-text

Estabrooks, C. A. (1998). Will evidence-based nursing practice make practice perfect? *Canadian Journal of Nursing Research, 30*(1), 15-36.

Grady, P. A. (2010). Translational research and nursing science. *Nursing Outlook, 58,* 164-166. Doi: 10.1016/j.outlook.2010.01.001.

Horsley, J., Crane, J., & Bingle, J. (1978). Research utilization as an organizational process. *Journal of Nursing Administration, 8*(7), 4-6.

Horsley, J. A., Crane, J., Crabtree, M. K., & Wood, D. J. (1983). *Using research to improve nursing practice.* New York: Grune & Stratton.

Institute of Medicine (IOM). (2001). *Crossing the quality chasm: A new health system for the 21st century.* Washington, DC: The National Academies Press.

Institute of Medicine (IOM). (2003). *Health professions education: A bridge to quality.* Washington, DC: The National Academies Press.

Institute of Medicine (IOM). (2010). *The future of nursing: Leading change, advancing health.* Washington, DC: The National Academies Press.

Krueger, J. C. (1978). Utilization of nursing research: The planning process. *Journal of Nursing Administration, 8*(1), 6-9.

McQueen, L., & McCormick, K. A. (2001). Translating evidence into practice: Guidelines and automated implementation tools. In, V. K. Saba & K. A. McCormick (Eds.), *Essentials of Computers for Nurses: Informatics for the New Millennium* (pp. 335-356). New York: McGraw Hill Publishers.

National Library of Medicine. (2011).Retrieved from: http://www.nlm.nih.gov/bsd/index_stats_comp.html

Newhouse, R. P., Dearholt, S., Poe, S., Pugh, L. C., & White, K. (2007). Organizational change strategies for evidence-based practice. *Journal of Nursing Administration, 37*(12), 552-557.

Pronovost, P. J. (2010). Learning accountability for patient outcomes. *JAMA, 304(2),* 204-205. doi: 10.1001/jama.2010.979.

Shin, J. H., Haynes, R. B., & Johnston, M. E. (1993). Effect of problem-based, self-directed education on life-long learning. *Canadian Medical Association Journal, 148*(6), 969-976.

Titler, M. G. (2004). Methods in translation science. *Worldviews on Evidence-based Nursing, 1*(1), 38-48.

Weaver, C., Warren, J. J., & Delaney, C. (2005). Bedside, classroom and bench: Collaborative strategies to generate evidence-based knowledge for nursing practice. *International Journal of Medical Informatics, 74*(11-12), 989-999.

Zerhouni, E. (2006). Research funding. NIH in the post doubling era: Realities and strategies. *Science, 314*(5802), 1088-1090.

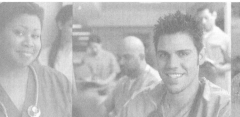
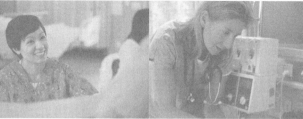

2

Critical Thinking and Evidence-Based Practice

Anne E. Belcher, PhD, RN, AOCN, ANEF, FAAN

Zeina E. Khouri-Stevens, PhD, RN

The nature of nursing itself compels nurses to play an active role in advancing best practices in patient care. Professional nursing practice involves making judgments; without judgments, nursing is merely technical work (Coles, 2002). Professional judgment is enabled by critical thinking. Critical thinking has many definitions in the literature; however, the complexity of the process requires not only definition, but also explanation (Riddell, 2007).

Paul and Elder (2005) define critical thinking as a skill that enables a person to think regularly at a higher level. It transforms thinking in two directions, increasing it systematically and comprehensively. Critical thinking is a complex cognitive process of questioning, seeking information, analyzing, synthesizing, drawing conclusions from available information, and transforming knowledge into action (AACN, 2008; Scheffer & Rubenfeld, 2006). It is a dynamic process, foundational for clinical reasoning and decision-making, and, as such, is an essential component for evidence-based practice (EBP). Every clinical scenario gives the nurse an opportunity to use acquired knowledge and skills to care effectively for the particular individual, family, or group (Dickerson, 2005). Regardless of the nature or source of evidence relating to patient care, critical thinking supplies the necessary skills and cognitive habits needed to support EBP (Profetto-McGrath, 2005).

Heaslip (2008) clearly articulates the importance of critical thinking in en-suring safe nursing practice and quality care: "Critical thinking when developed in the practitioner includes adherence to intellectual standards, proficiency in using reasoning, a commitment to develop and maintain intellectual traits of the mind and habits of thought and the competent use of thinking skills and abili-ties for sound clinical judgments and safe decision-making" (p. 834). She further describes what it means to think like a nurse: "To think like a nurse requires that we learn the content of nursing: the ideas, concepts, and theories of nursing and develop our intellectual capacities and skills so that we become disciplined, self-directed, critical thinkers" (p. 1).

This chapter describes the knowledge and skills needed to foster critical thinking and has the following objectives:

- Illustrate the similarities between EBP and the nursing process
- Differentiate among critical thinking, reasoning, reflection, and judgment
- Describe how these skills influence evidence appraisal and decisions about applying evidence to practice
- Discuss the role of critical thinking in the Practice question, Evidence, and Translation (PET) process

Evidence-Based Practice and the Nursing Process

EBP and what constitutes evidence is continually evolving. Nurses, key members of interprofessional teams, participate meaningfully in translating best practices to patient care. Nursing skills that may need strengthening, however, are posing answerable questions, gathering and critically appraising evidence, and determin-ing whether or how to translate relevant findings into practice. These skills are prerequisites to informed decision-making and the application of best practices to the care of patients.

The American Nurses Association (ANA) *Nursing: Scope and Standards of Practice* (2010) references each step of the nursing process, from collection of comprehensive data pertinent to the patient's health or illness through evaluation of the outcomes of planned interventions. It also references integration of the best available evidence, including research findings, to guide practice decisions.

The similarity between EBP and the nursing process is evident; both are problem-solving strategies. The nursing process structures practice through the following problem-solving stages: assessment, diagnosis, outcome identification, planning, intervention, and evaluation. Although critical thinking is generally considered inherent in the nursing process, this has not been empirically demonstrated (Fesler-Birch, 2005). Nevertheless, the nursing process does require certain skills that are also necessary for critical thinking, such as seeking information and synthesizing it (assessment), drawing conclusions from available information (diagnosis), and transforming knowledge into a plan of action (planning). However, the concept of critical thinking extends beyond this well-defined process.

The Johns Hopkins Nursing Evidence-based Practice (JHNEBP) Model's Practice question, Evidence, and Translation (PET) process structures the activities of EBP. The nurse asks a focused practice question (P), searches for and appraises relevant evidence (E), and translates the evidence into patient care and evaluates the outcome (T). Each phase requires an analogous set of critical thinking skills including questioning, information seeking, synthesizing, logical reasoning, and transforming knowledge.

Carper (1978) defined four patterns of knowing in nursing: empirical (the science of nursing), ethical (the code of nursing), personal (knowledge gained from interpersonal relationships between the nurse and the patient), and aesthetic (the art of nursing). Each of these patterns contributes to the body of evidence on which practice is based. Building on Carper's work, McKenna, Cutcliffe, and McKenna (2000) postulated four types of evidence to consider:

- **Empirical:** Based on scientific research
- **Ethical:** Based on the nurse's knowledge of and respect for the patient's values and preferences

- **Personal:** Based on the nurse's experience in caring for the individual patient
- **Aesthetic:** Based on the nurse's intuition, interpretation, understanding, and personal values

It is the compilation and critical appraisal of all types of evidence, alone and as they relate to each other, that results in the nurse's decision to adopt or reject evidence for use in the care of the individual patient.

The JHNEBP Model broadly categorizes evidence as either research or non-research. Scientific (empirical) findings comprise research evidence, whereas non-research evidence includes ethical, personal, and aesthetic evidence. Inherent in the JHNEBP Model is the relationship between critical thinking and the judicious application of evidence in practice through the PET process.

Critical Thinking, Reasoning, Reflection, and Judgment

Contemporary nurses are at risk of becoming increasingly task-focused as a result of multiple new technologies and the shift to electronic documentation and health records. Task-focused practice is expected for newly graduated nurses. However, this focus precludes reflection on the who, what, where, when, and why of care. Even experienced nurses may fail to ask *why* as they become immersed in managing the diverse and now ever-present technology. EBP not only directs nurses to ask *why*, but also guides them in answering questions and making patient-care decisions.

The growing complexity and intensity of patient care demands multiple "higher order" thinking strategies that include not only critical thinking, but also critical reasoning, reflection, and judgment (Benner, Hughes, & Sutphen, 2008, pp. 1-88; see Box 2.1.) Each of these concepts and its applicability to EBP is discussed below.

Box 2.1	Definitions of Critical Thinking, Reasoning, Reflection, and Judgment
Concept	**Definition**
Critical thinking	Ability to make inferences explicit, along with the assumptions or premises upon which those inferences are based
Reasoning	Drawing conclusions or inferences from observations, facts, or hypotheses
Reflection	Ability to create and clarify the meaning of a particular experience
Judgment	Act of judging or deciding on the basis of reason, evidence, logic, and good sense

While critical thinkers strive to develop the ability to make their inferences explicit, along with the assumptions or premises upon which those inferences are based, nurses who employ *reasoning* draw conclusions or inferences from observations, facts, or hypotheses. All reasoning has a purpose; it attempts to figure something out, settle a question, or solve a problem. Reasoning is based on assumptions from a specific point of view and on data, information, and evidence expressed through, and shaped by, concepts and ideas. The inferences or interpretations by which one draws conclusions and gives meaning to data have implications and consequences (Paul & Elder, 2005).

Reflection, a key cognitive mechanism in critical thinking, enables nurses to create and clarify the meaning of a particular experience (Forneris & Peden-McAlpine, 2007). Reflection in the context of nursing practice "is viewed as a process of transforming unconscious types of knowledge and practices into conscious, explicit, and logically articulated knowledge and practice that allows for transparent and justifiable clinical decision-making" (Mantzoukas, 2007, p. 7).

Judgment reflects the act of judging or deciding. People have good judgment when they decide on the basis of understanding and good sense. Forming an opinion or belief, deciding, or acting on a decision is done on the basis of implicit or explicit judgments. To cultivate the ability to think critically, nurses have to develop the habit of judging on the basis of reason, evidence, logic, and good sense (http://www.criticalthinking.org).

Nursing Expertise, Intellectual Competence, and Evidence-Based Practice

In her landmark book, *From Novice to Expert: Excellence and Power in Clinical Nursing Practice*, Benner (2001) applied the Dreyfus Model of Skill Acquisition (Dreyfus & Dreyfus, 1986) to the professional development of nurses. Progressing through the stages of novice to expert, nurses learn to link technical expertise with intuitive expertise. That is, to manage patient-care situations, nurses refine their critical thinking skills to integrate experience with acquired knowledge. Hawkins, Elder, and Paul (2010, pp. 11-12) suggest thinking critically requires having command of universal intellectual standards:

- **Clarity:** Elaborating on issues or giving an example
- **Accuracy:** Checking facts; determining if facts are true
- **Precision:** Providing additional details
- **Relevance:** Correlating evidence to the issue at hand
- **Depth:** Accounting for complexities in a particular situation
- **Breadth:** Considering alternatives to the most apparent solutions
- **Logic:** Judging whether an action is prudent given the circumstances
- **Significance:** Determining the most important problem to consider
- **Fairness:** Equitably representing other viewpoints

These intellectual standards "must be applied to thinking whenever one is interested in checking the quality of reasoning about a problem, issue, or situation" (p. 7). Such intellectual rigor is invaluable to members of the EBP team. If a statement is unclear, the team cannot judge its accuracy or relevance to the practice question. Similarly, superficial answers, or those that present only one point of view, do not address the complexities of most patient care questions. Finally, after developing a well-reasoned, evidence-based answer, the team members must decide on the feasibility of translating the answer into practice for the particular patient population.

Nursing, in particular, requires specific cognitive skills for excellence in practice; developing these is an essential aspect of their nursing education (Taylor-Seehafer, Abel, Tyler, & Sonstein, 2004). Cognitive skills include the following:

- **Divergent thinking:** The ability to analyze a variety of opinions
- **Reasoning:** The ability to differentiate between fact and conjecture
- **Reflection:** Time to deliberate and identify multidimensional processes
- **Creativity:** Considering multiple solutions
- **Clarification:** Noting similarities, differences, and assumptions
- **Basic support:** Evaluating credibility of sources of information

Beyond the requisite nursing knowledge and skills, practitioners must have the necessary attitudes, attributes, and habits of mind to use this knowledge appropriately and to complement these skills effectively (Profetto-McGrath, 2005). One approach to defining these dispositions is based on the proposition that certain *intellectual virtues* are valuable to the critical thinker (Foundation for Critical Thinking, 1996). In a second approach, *habits of the mind* are identified and exhibited by critical thinkers (Scheffer & Rubenfeld, 2006). These two complementary disposition sets are outlined in Table 2.1. When participating in EBP projects, the team should be aware of these intellectual virtues and habits to avoid the pitfalls of vague, fragmented, or closed-minded thinking.

Table 2.1   Attributes of Critical Thinkers

Intellectual Virtues of Critical Thinkers	Habits of Mind of Critical Thinkers
Intellectual Humility: Being aware of the limits of one's knowledge	Confidence: Assurance of one's own ability to reason
Intellectual Courage: Being open and fair when addressing ideas, viewpoints, or beliefs that differ from one's own	Contextual Perspective: Ability to consider the whole in its entirety
Intellectual Empathy: Being aware of the need to put one's self in another's place to achieve genuine understanding	Creativity: Intellectual inventiveness

Table 2.1   Attributes of Critical Thinkers (continued)

Intellectual Virtues of Critical Thinkers	Habits of Mind of Critical Thinkers
Intellectual Integrity: Holding one's self to the same rigorous standards of evidence and proof as one does others	Flexibility: Capacity to adapt
Intellectual Perseverance: Being cognizant of the need to use rational principles despite obstacles to doing so	Inquisitiveness: Seeking knowledge and understanding through thoughtful questioning and observation
Faith in Reason: Being confident that people can learn to critically think for themselves	Intellectual Integrity: Seeking the truth, even if results are contrary to one's assumptions or beliefs
Fair-mindedness: Understanding that one needs to treat all viewpoints in an unbiased fashion	Intuition: Sense of knowing without conscious use of reason
	Open-mindedness: Receptivity to divergent views
	Perseverance: Determination to stay on course
	Reflection: Contemplation for a deeper understanding and self-evaluation

Educating for Critical Thinking Skills

Cultivating critical thinking skills in nursing students and practicing nurses at all levels is a primary goal for nurse educators and nurse administrators (Eisenhauer, Hurley, & Dolan, 2007). Most educators would agree that learning to think critically is among the most desirable goals of formal schooling (Abrami et al., 2008). "This includes not only thinking about important problems within a specific disciplinary area, but also thinking about the social, political, and ethical challenges of everyday life in a multifaceted and increasingly complex world" (p. 1102). Because of the unpredictable nature of patient care, nurses need the ability to analyze and interpret cues, weigh evidence, and respond appropriately and promptly to changing clinical situations, especially those requiring immediate action. Furthermore, the ability to think critically is an essential competency for EBP teams when evaluating the cumulative body of evidence for its potential applicability to particular patient care situations.

Educators can use diverse approaches to structure orientation and training for newly hired nurses, whether experienced or newly graduated. Multiple orientation models can be found in the literature. Educators using the Benner model, From Novice to Expert, as a framework, may ask: "At what stage would teaching critical thinking and the importance of evidence-based practice be appropriate?" and "When would introducing such skills yield results and benefits for the new nurse/orientee?" The literature suggests that teaching critical thinking and acquiring these skills is best done following the novice stage of development because in the novice stage, nurses are still mastering simple tasks and step-by-step procedures. Analysis and reflection, critical-thinking skills needed for evidence-based practice, develop during later stages in Benner's model. It is true that these and other critical-thinking skills may increase inquisitiveness, questioning of practice, and inquiry as to the best way to apply new knowledge. Nevertheless, it may be best to only *introduce* staff to the concepts of critical thinking and EBP and *set expectations* for using them at the advanced-beginner or proficient stage of Benner's model. Encouraging nurses to ask questions allows them to approach their day-to-day care with a clearer understanding and a view to improving that care, which leads naturally to the PET process.

Critical Thinking and the PET Process

Applying evidence in practice requires a number of steps. The role of critical thinking in each phase of the Practice question, Evidence, and Translation (PET) process is described in this section.

Critical Thinking in Posing the Practice Question

In the PET process, the EBP team first defines the scope of the problem by considering the entire situation including the background and environment relevant to the phenomenon of interest. During this activity, interprofessional team members apply intellectual habits such as confidence, creativity, flexibility, inquisitiveness, intellectual integrity, and open-mindedness. Posing an answerable practice question determines what information to seek and the direction in which to search. Creating a well-built question often can be more challenging than actually answering the question (Schlosser, Koul, & Costello, 2007). The universal intellectual standards cited in the prior section of this chapter can assist the team in determining the quality of reasoning about a problem, issue, or situation (Paul & Elder, 1996b) and can help refine the practice question by making it clear, accurate, precise, and relevant. If the question posed is unclear or is based on false assumptions, it may not be truly reflective of the issue of concern. If the question is nonspecific, it may not contain sufficient detail to be answerable. If it is irrelevant to the concern, it could lead to evidence that does not help provide an appropriate answer. The practice question should have enough depth and breadth to reflect the complexities of care, but not be so broad that the search for evidence becomes too difficult to manage.

Schlosser, Koul, and Costello (2007) proposed identifying and formalizing the process of asking well-built questions to distinguish them from poorly stated questions. The JHNEBP Model uses a Question Development Tool (see Appendix B) to serve as a guide for defining the scope of the problem and generating useful questions. Components of this tool as they relate to critical thinking standards are outlined in Table 2.2. The Patient, Intervention, Comparison, and Outcome (PICO) organizing template (Richardson, Wilson, Nishikawa, & Hayward, 1995) can be used to structure question development and is discussed in more detail in Chapter 4.

Table 2.2   Practice Question Development and Critical Thinking Standards

Practice Question Components	Critical Thinking Standards and Questions
What is the practice issue? What is the current practice?	Clarity: Is the issue clear? Can we give an example?
How was the practice issue identified?	Accuracy: What evidence (quantitative or qualitative) supports the issue or problem? What methods were used to verify the truth of evidence?

Practice Question Components	Critical Thinking Standards and Questions
What are the PICO components? (patient/population/problem, intervention, comparison with other treatments if applicable, outcome)	Precision: Can we provide more detail on the issue? What is the issue? What interventions are we questioning? Do we want to compare this with some other intervention?
	Logic: What is our desired outcome? Does it really make sense?
State the search question in narrow, manageable terms.	Precision: Can we be more specific?
What evidence must be gathered?	Relevance: How is this evidence connected to the question? Are we addressing the most significant factors related to the question?
State the search strategy, database, and keywords.	Breadth: Do we need to consider other points of view? Are there other ways to look at the question?

Critical Thinking and Appraising Evidence

The evidence phase of the PET process requires proficiency in the following critical thinking skills: seeking information, analyzing, interpreting, and drawing conclusions from available information. The critical analysis, synthesis, and interpretation of evidence are made explicit by the use of rating scales. These standardized levels of evidence facilitate differentiating among varying strengths and quality of evidence. The underlying assumption is that recommendations from strong evidence of high quality would be more likely to represent best practices than evidence of lower strength and lesser quality. The rating scale used in the JHNEBP Model to determine strength of evidence is found in Appendix C.

Research evidence is generally given a higher strength rating than is non-research evidence, in particular when the scientific evidence is of high quality. Nurses on EBP teams apply critical-thinking skills when appraising scientific research by focusing on two major components: study design (usually classified as experimental, quasi-experimental, nonexperimental, and qualitative) and study quality (evaluation of study methods and procedure). When evaluating the summary of overall evidence, nurses consider four major components: study design, quality, consistency (similarities in the size and/or direction of estimated effects across studies), and directness (the extent to which subjects, interventions, and outcome measures are similar to those of interest) (GRADE Working Group, 2004). The various types of research evidence and their associated levels of evidential strength are further explored in Chapter 6.

Because of the complex human and environmental context of patient care, research evidence is not sufficient to inform practice. In many instances, scientific evidence either does not exist or is insufficient to shape nursing practice for the individual patient, population, or system. Non-research evidence also is needed to inform nursing knowledge and generally includes summaries of research evidence reports, expert opinion, practitioner experience and expertise, patient preferences, and human/organizational experience. Clinical appraisal of the strength of non-research evidence is not as well established as is that for scientific evidence and is, therefore, more challenging. Because non-research evidence is thought to be outside the realm of science, and thus less meaningful, appraisal methods have rarely been considered. The various types of non-research evidence are discussed in Chapter 7.

The development of any EBP skill set is an evolutionary process. Critical thinking is thought by many to be "a lifelong process requiring self-awareness, knowledge, and practice" (Brunt, 2005). The JHNEBP Model uses a broadly defined quality rating scale to provide structure, yet allows for the application of critical thinking skills specific to the knowledge and experience of the team reviewing the evidence. This scale can accommodate qualitative judgments related both to scientific and non-research evidence.

Judgments of quality should be continually approached in relative terms. The EBP team assigns a quality grade for each piece of evidence reviewed. The judgment that underlies this determination is in relation to the body of past and present evidence that each member has reviewed. As the group and its individual members gain experience reading and appraising research, their abilities and judgments will likely improve.

Critical Thinking and Translation

The challenge for a nurse participating in an EBP project is translating the contributions of each type of evidence to patient care decisions. Not only must the team grade the strength and quality of evidence, but they must also determine the compatibility of recommendations with the patient's values and preferences and the clinician's expertise (Melnyk & Fineout-Overholt, 2006).

Two goals of critical thinking are to assess credibility of information and to work through problems to make the best decisions (Halpern, 1996). This requires flexibility, persistence, and self-awareness. It challenges nurses to consider alternate ways of thinking and acting. Maudsley and Strivens (2000) postulated that a competent practitioner must use critical thinking skills to appraise evidence, tempering realistic notions of scientific evidence with a healthy dose of reflective skepticism. This certainly holds true for nurses as they execute the translation phase of evidence-based practice.

Recommendations for Nurse Leaders

Though some key elements of critical thinking are not discussed within the context of the nursing process, some components of critical thinking are clearly vital to the work of nursing. Therefore, nursing accreditation bodies recognize critical thinking as "a significant outcome for graduates at the baccalaureate and master's levels" (Ali, Bantz, & Siktberg, 2005). Furthermore, critical thinking skills such as questioning, analyzing, synthesizing, and drawing conclusions from available information are definite assets to the nurse in reaching meaningful evidence-based practice decisions.

Senge (1990) described team learning—the interaction of a team to produce learning and solve problems—as an essential component of learning organizations in which leaders continuously develop capacity for the future. Building capacity for nurses to carry out EBP projects is of strategic importance for nurse leaders; ensuring nurses have the knowledge and skills required to procure and judge the value of evidence is a top leadership priority.

One way to achieve the successful cultural transition to evidence-based practice is to apply the notion of interactive team learning (Sams, Penn, & Facteau,

2004). As members of the EBP team gain experience reviewing and critiquing both research and non-research evidence related to a clinical question, their motivation to integrate evidence into practice will increase. Thus, nurses need to have a sound knowledge base regarding the nature of research and non-research evidence.

Nurse leaders can best support EBP by providing clinicians with the knowledge and skills necessary to pose answerable questions, to seek and appraise scientific and other quantitative and qualitative evidence within the context of non-research evidence, and to make a determination on the advisability of translating evidence into practice. Only through continuous learning and experience can clinicians gain the confidence needed to incorporate the broad range of evidence into the development of protocols and care standards and into the personalized care of the individual patient. Nurse educators also can advance EBP by including related skill development as part of nursing curricula. This can provide a larger pool from which nurse leaders can draw potential employees with a strong educational background in EBP.

Summary

In today's dynamic health care environment, nurses cannot achieve expertise without maintaining continual awareness of the entire realm of known research. It is virtually impossible for staff nurses to give their complete attention to keeping track of all studies relevant to their practice. Knowledge gained through professional education, coupled with non-research learning, guides much of the nurse's practice.

Valid clinical questions arise during the course of the nurse's day-to-day patient care activities. These are the questions that form the basis for many EBP projects and that benefit from the combined critical thinking of collaborative teams of nurses and their interprofessional colleagues. As Scheffer and Rubenfeld (2006) eloquently stated, "Putting the critical thinking dimensions into the development of evidence-based practice competency demonstrates how critical thinking can be taken out of the toolbox and used in the real world" (p. 195).

References

Abrami, P. C., Bernard, R. M., Borokhovski, E., Wade, A., Surkes, M. A., Tamim, R., & Zhang, D. (2008). Instructional interventions affecting critical thinking skills and dispositions: A stage 1 meta-analysis. *Review of Educational Research, 78*(4), 1102-1134.

Ali, N. S., Bantz, D. & Siktberg, L. (2005). Validation of critical thinking skills in online responses. *Journal of Nursing Education, 44*(2), 90-94.

American Association of Colleges of Nursing (AACN). (2008). The essentials of baccalaureate education for professional nursing practice. Washington, DC: AACN.

American Nurses Association (ANA). (2010). *Nursing: Scope and standards of practice.* Washington, DC: ANA.

Benner, P. E. (2001). *From novice to expert: Excellence and power in clinical nursing practice.* (Commemorative edition). Upper Saddle River, NJ: Prentice Hall.

Benner, P., Hughes, R. G., & Sutphen, M. (2008). Clinical reasoning, decision making, and action: Thinking critically and clinically. In R. G. Hughes (Ed.), *Patient safety and quality: An evidence-based handbook for nurses.* (Prepared with support from the Robert Wood Johnson Foundation.) AHRQ Publication No. 08-0043. Rockville: MD: Agency for healthcare Research and Quality, April 2008.

Brunt, B. A. (2005). Critical thinking in nursing: An integrated review. *The Journal of Continuing Education in Nursing, 36*(2), 60-67.

Carper, B. (1978). Fundamental patterns of knowing in nursing. *Advances in Nursing Science, 1*(1), 13-23.

Coles, C. (2002). Developing professional judgment. *Journal of Continuing Education, 22*(1), 3-10.

Dickerson, P. S. (2005). Nurturing critical thinkers. *The Journal of Continuing Education in Nursing, 36*(2), 68-72.

Dreyfus, H. L., & Dreyfus, S. E. (1986). *Mind over machine*. New York, NY: The Free Press.

Eisenhauer, L. A., Hurley, A. C., & Dolan, N. (2007). Nurses' reported thinking during medication administration. *Journal of Nursing Scholarship, 39*(1), 82-87.

Fesler-Birch, D. M. (2005). Critical thinking and patient outcomes: A review. *Nursing Outlook, 53*(2), 59-65.

Forneris, S. G., & Peden-McAlpine, C. (2007). Evaluation of a reflective learning intervention to improve critical thinking in novice nurses. *Journal of Advanced Nursing, 57*(4), 410-421.

Foundation for Critical Thinking. (1996). Valuable intellectual virtues. Retrieved from http://criticalthinking.org/resources/articles/

GRADE Working Group (2004). Grading quality of evidence and strength of recommendations. *British Medical Journal, 328*(7454), 1490-1498.

Halpern, D. F. (1996). *Thought and knowledge: An introduction to critical thinking.* Mahwah, NJ: Erlbaun.

Hawkins, D., Elder, L., & Paul, R. (2010). *The thinker's guide to clinical reasoning.* Foundation for Critical Thinking Press.

Heaslip, P. (2008). Critical thinking: To think like a nurse. Retrieved from http://www.criticalthinking.org/pages/critical-thinking-and-nursing/834.

Mantzoukas, S. (2007). A review of evidence-based practice, nursing research, and reflection: Leveling the hierarchy. *Journal of Clinical Nursing* (Online Early Articles) 214-223.

Maudsley, G., & Strivens, J. (2000). 'Science,' 'critical thinking', and 'competence' for tomorrow's doctors. A review of terms and concepts. *Medical Education, 34*(1), 53-60.

McKenna, H., Cutcliffe, J., & McKenna, P. (2000). Evidence-based practice: Demolishing some myths. *Nursing Standard, 14*(16), 39-42.

Melnyk, B. M., & Fineout-Overholt, E. (2006). Consumer preferences and values as an integral key to evidence-based practice. *Nursing Administration Quarterly, 30*(2), 123-127.

Paul, R., & Elder, L. (1996b). The critical mind is a questioning mind. Retrieved from http://criticalthinking.org/resources/articles/

Paul, R., & Elder, L. (2005). *The miniature guide to critical thinking: Concepts and tools.* Dillon Beach, CA: The Foundation for Critical Thinking.

Profetto-McGrath, J. (2005). Critical thinking and evidence-based practice. *Journal of Professional Nursing, 21*(6), 364-371.

Richardson, W. S., Wilson, M. C., Nishikawa, J., & Hayward, R. S. (1995). The well-built clinical question: A key to evidence-based decisions. *ACP Journal Club, 123*(3), A12-A13.

Riddell, T. (2007). Critical assumptions: Thinking critically about critical thinking. *Journal of Nursing Education, 46*(3), 121-126.

Sams, L., Penn, B. K., & Facteau, L. (2004). The challenge of using evidence-based practice. *Journal of Nursing Administration, 34*(9), 407-414.

Scheffer, B. K., & Rubenfeld, M. G. (2006). Critical thinking: A tool in search of a job. *Journal of Nursing Education, 45*(6), 195-196.

Schlosser, R. W., Koul, R., & Costello, J. (2007). Asking well-built questions for evidence-based practice in augmentative and alternative communication. *Journal of Communication Disorders, 40*(3), 225-238.

Senge, P. M. (1990). *The fifth discipline: The art and practice of the learning organization.* New York: Doubleday.

Taylor-Seehafer, M. A., Abel, E., Tyler, D. O., & Sonstein, F. C. (2004). Integrating evidence-based practice in nurse practitioner education. *Journal of the American Academy of Nurse Practitioners, 16*(12), 520-525.

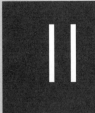

The Johns Hopkins Nursing Evidence-Based Practice Model and Guidelines

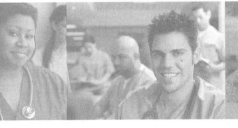

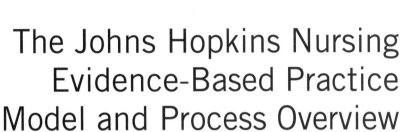

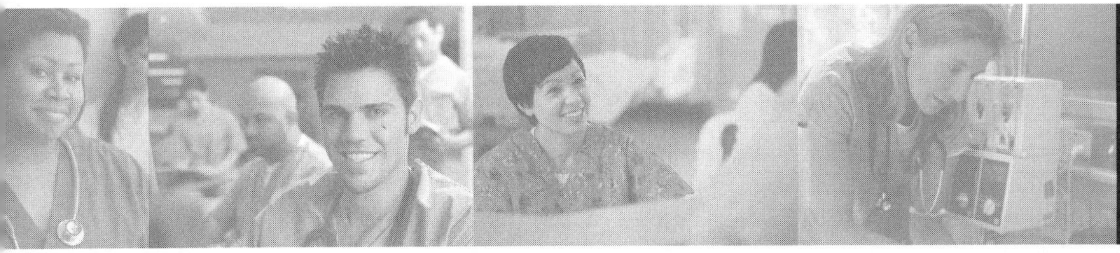

3

The Johns Hopkins Nursing Evidence-Based Practice Model and Process Overview

Sandra L. Dearholt, MS, RN

Evidence-based practice (EBP) is now a core competency for all health care professionals (IOM, 2003). This requires leaders in both academia and service to align their educational and practice environments to promote practice based on evidence, to cultivate a spirit of continuous inquiry, and to translate the highest quality evidence into practice. Selecting a model for EBP fosters end-user adoption of evidence and embeds this practice into the fabric of the organization. The objectives for this chapter are to:

- Describe The Johns Hopkins Nursing Evidence-based Practice Model
- Introduce bedside nurses and nurse leaders to the PET process (Practice Question, Evidence, and Translation), a tool to guide nurses through the steps in applying EBP

The Johns Hopkins Nursing Evidence-Based Practice Model

The Johns Hopkins Nursing Evidence-Based Practice Model (JHNEBP; see Figure 3.1) depicts three essential cornerstones that are the foundation for professional nursing: practice, education, and research.

- *Practice,* the basic component of all nursing activity (Porter-O'Grady, 1984), reflects the translation of what nurses know into what they do. It is the who, what, when, where, why, and how that addresses the range of nursing activities that define the care a patient receives (American Nurses Association [ANA], 2010). It is an integral component of health care organizations.

- *Education* reflects the acquisition of nursing knowledge and skills necessary to build expertise and maintain competency.

- *Research* generates new knowledge for the profession and enables the development of practices based on scientific evidence. Nurses not only "rely on this evidence to guide their policies and practices, but also as a way of quantifying the nurses' impact on the health outcomes of healthcare consumers" (American Nurses Association, 2010, p. 22).

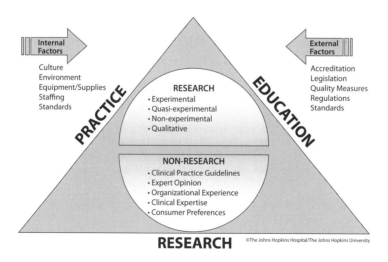

Figure 3.1   The Johns Hopkins Nursing Evidence-Based Practice Model

Nursing Practice

Nurses are bound by, and held to, standards established by professional nursing organizations. For example, the American Nurses Association (2010) has identified six standards of nursing practice (scope) that are based on the nursing process (see Table 3.1) and ten standards of professional performance (see Table 3.2). In addition to the ANA, professional specialty nursing organizations establish standards of care for specific patient populations. Collectively, these standards define scope of practice, set expectations for evaluating performance, and guide the care provided to patients and families. Because these standards provide broad expectations for practice, all settings where health care is delivered must translate these expectations into organization-specific policies, protocols, and procedures. As part of this process, nurses need to question the basis of their practice and use an evidence-based approach to validate or change current practice based on the evidence. Conventionally, nurses have based their practice on policies, protocols, and procedures often unsubstantiated by evidence (Melnyk, Finout-Overholt, Stillwell, & Williamson, 2009). The use of an evidence-based approach, however, is now the standard set by professional nursing organizations and is an essential component of the Magnet Model for organizations aspiring to Magnet recognition (Reigle et al., 2008).

The Magnet Model (see Figure 3.2) has five key components: (a) transformational leadership; (b) structural empowerment; (c) exemplary professional practice; (d) new knowledge, innovations, and improvements; and (e) empirical outcomes. To provide *transformational leadership*, nursing leaders need to have vision, influence, clinical knowledge, and expertise (Wolf, Triolo & Ponte, 2008). They need to create the vision and the environment that supports EBP activities, such as continuous questioning of nursing practice, translation of existing knowledge, and development of new knowledge. Through *structural empowerment* nursing leaders promote professional staff involvement and autonomy in identifying best practices and using the EBP process to change practice. Magnet organizations demonstrate *exemplary professional practice* such as maintaining strong professional practice models; partnering with patients, families, and interprofessional team members; and focusing on systems that promote patient and staff safety. *New knowledge, innovations, and improvements* challenge Magnet organizations to design new models of care, apply existing and new evidence to practice, and make visible contributions to the science of nursing (American Nurses Credentialing Center [ANCC], 2011). Additionally, organizations are required to have a heightened focus on *empirical outcomes* to evaluate quality. The EBP process supports the use of data sources such as quality improvement results, financial analysis, and program evaluations when answering EBP questions.

Table 3.1   American Nurses Association Standards of Practice

1. *Assessment:* The collection of comprehensive data pertinent to the health care consumer's health and/or situation. Data collection should be systematic and ongoing. As applicable, evidence-based assessment tools or instruments should be used, for example, evidence-based fall assessment tools, pain rating scales, or wound assessment tools.

2. *Diagnosis:* The analysis of assessment data to determine the diagnoses or issues.

3. *Outcomes identification:* The identification of expected outcomes for a plan individualized to the health care consumer or the situation. Associated risks, benefits, costs, current scientific evidence, expected trajectory of the condition, and clinical expertise should be considered when formulating expected outcomes.

4. *Planning:* The development of a plan that prescribes strategies and alternatives to attain expected outcomes. The plan integrates current scientific evidence, trends, and research.

5. *Implementation:* Implementation of the identified plan, which includes partnering with the person, family, significant other, and caregivers as appropriate to implement the plan in a safe, realistic, and timely manner. Utilizes evidence-based interventions and treatments specific to the diagnosis or problem.

   a. Coordination of Care: Coordinates/organizes and documents the plan of care.

   b. Health Teaching and Health Promotion: Employing strategies to promote health and a healthy environment.

   c. Consultation: Graduate-level prepared specialty nurse or advanced practice registered nurse provides consultation to influence the identified plan, enhance the abilities of others, and effect change.

   d. Prescriptive Authority and Treatment: Advanced practice registered nurse prescribes evidence-based treatments, therapies, and procedures considering the health care consumer's comprehensive health care needs.

6. *Evaluation:* Progress towards attainment of outcomes. Includes conducting a systematic, ongoing, and criterion-based evaluation of the outcomes in relation to the structures and processes prescribed by the plan of care and the indicated timeline.

Table 3.2   American Nurses Association Standards of Professional Performance

1. *Ethics:* The delivery of care in a manner that preserves and protects health care consumer autonomy, dignity, rights, values, and beliefs.

2. *Education:* Attaining knowledge and competency that reflects current nursing practice. Participation in ongoing educational activities. Commitment to lifelong learning through self-reflection and inquiry to address learning and personal growth needs.

3. *Evidence-Based Practice and Research:* The integration of evidence and research findings into practice by utilizing current evidence-based knowledge, including research findings, to guide practice.

4. *Quality of Practice:* Contributing to quality nursing practice through quality improvement activities, documenting the nursing process in a responsible, accountable, and ethical manner, and using creativity and innovation to enhance nursing care.

5. *Communication:* Communicating effectively in a variety of formats in all areas of practice.

6. *Leadership:* Providing leadership in the professional practice setting and the profession.

7. *Collaboration:* Collaboration with health care consumer, family, and others in the conduct of nursing practice.

8. *Professional Practice Evaluation:* Evaluation of one's nursing practice in relation to professional practice standards and guidelines, relevant statutes, rules, and regulations.

9. *Resource Utilization:* Utilizes appropriate resources to plan and provide nursing services that are safe, effective, and financially responsible.

10. *Environmental Health:* Practicing in a safe and environmentally safe and healthy manner. Utilizes scientific evidence to determine if a product or treatment is an environmental threat.

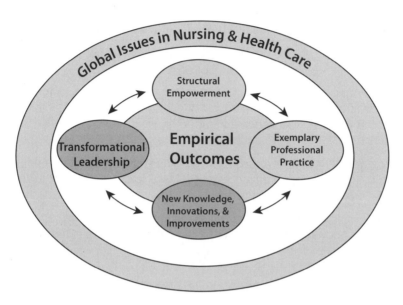

Figure 3.2   American Nurses Credentialing Center Magnet Model Components

An organization's ability to create opportunities for nurses, as part of an interprofessional team, to develop EBP questions, evaluate evidence, promote critical thinking, make practice changes, and promote professional development has a major impact on achieving Magnet status. Anecdotal evidence suggests nursing staff who participate in the EBP process feel a greater sense of empowerment and satisfaction as a result of contributing to changes in nursing practice based on evidence. Change may also be more readily accepted within the organization and by other disciplines when it is based on evidence that has been evaluated through an interprofessional EBP process.

Nursing Education

Nursing education begins with basic education (generally an associate or a bachelor's degree) in which fundamental nursing skills and knowledge, natural and behavioral sciences, professional values, behaviors, and attitudes are learned. Advanced education (a master's or doctorate degree) expands knowledge based on theory, refines practice, and often leads to specialization in a particular practice area. Advanced nursing education incorporates an increased emphasis on the application of research and other types of evidence to influence or change nursing practice and care delivery systems.

Ongoing education, such as conferences, seminars, workshops, and inservices, are required to remain current with new knowledge, technologies, and skills or to establish ongoing clinical competencies. Because the field of health care is becoming increasingly more complex and technical, no one individual can know everything about how best to provide safe and effective care, and no one degree can provide the necessary knowledge needed to span an entire career. It is, therefore, an essential expectation that nurses participate in lifelong learning and continued competency (IOM, 2011). Lifelong learning is not only individual learning, but also interprofessional, collaborative, and team-oriented learning. For example, using simulation and web training to educate nursing and medical students together on roles and responsibilities, effective communication, conflict resolution, and shared decision-making is expected to result in collaborative graduates ready to work effectively in patient-centered teams. Further, the use of interprofessional education is thought to foster collaboration in implementing policies, improving services, and preparing teams to solve problems that exceed the capacity of any one professional (IOM, 2011).

Nursing Research

Nursing research uses qualitative and quantitative systematic methods and an EBP approach directed toward the study and improvement of patient care, care systems, and therapeutic outcomes. Although it is commonly accepted that best practices are based on decisions validated by sound, scientific evidence, in fact, the rate at which current research is translated into nursing practice is often slow. Many nurses are influenced to some extent by what is known as *knowledge creep,* in which they gradually see the need to change practice based on limited research and word of mouth (Pape & Richards, 2010). Creating structures and support for nurses to use evidence in their clinical practice will help narrow this evidence-practice gap (Oman, Duran, & Fink, 2008). Nursing leaders need to support and encourage proficiency in and use of nursing research to generate new knowledge, inform practice, and promote quality patient outcomes. To accomplish this, the organization needs to build a strong infrastructure through the development of mentors, skills-building programs, financial support, computer access, and availability of research consultative services.

The JHNEBP Model—The Core

At the core of the Johns Hopkins Nursing EBP model is evidence. The sources of evidence include both research and non-research data which inform practice, education, and research. Research produces the strongest type of evidence to inform decisions about nursing practice. However, because research evidence answers a specific question under specific conditions, outcomes may not always be readily transferable to another clinical setting or patient population. Before translating research evidence into practice, nurses need to carefully consider the type of research, consistency of findings, quantity of supporting studies, quality of the studies, relevance of the findings to the clinical practice setting, and the benefits and risks of implementing the findings.

In many cases, research relevant to a particular nursing practice question may be limited. Consequently, nurses need to examine and evaluate other sources of non-research evidence, such as clinical guidelines, literature reviews, recommendations from national and local professional organizations, regulations, quality improvement data, and program evaluations. These, along with expert opinion, clinician judgment, and patient preferences, are sources of non-research evidence. Patient interviews, focus groups, and patient satisfaction surveys are all examples of preference-related evidence. Patients are taking a more active role in making decisions for their health care; therefore, clinicians need to discover what patients want, help them find accurate information, and support them in making these decisions (Krahn & Naglie, 2008). A patient's values, beliefs, and preferences will also influence the patient's desire to comply with treatments, despite the best evidence.

Internal and External Factors

The JHNEBP Model is an open system with interrelated components. As an open system, practice, education, and research are influenced not only by evidence, but also by external and internal factors. *External factors* can include accreditation bodies, legislation, quality measures, regulations, and standards. Accreditation bodies (e.g., The Joint Commission, Commission on Accreditation of Rehabilitation Facilities) require an organization to achieve and maintain high standards of practice and quality. Legislative and regulatory bodies (local, state, and federal) enact laws and regulations designed to protect the public and promote access to safe, quality health care services. Failure to follow these laws and regulations has adverse effects on an organization, most often financial. Examples of regulatory agencies include the Centers for Medicare and Medicaid Services, Food and Drug Administration, and state boards of nursing. State boards of nursing regulate nursing practice and enforce Nurse Practice Acts, which serves to protect the public. Quality measures (outcome and performance data) and professional standards serve as yardsticks for evaluating current practice and identifying areas for improvement or change. The American Nurses Credentialing Center, through its Magnet Recognition Program®, developed criteria to assess the quality of nursing and nursing excellence in organizations. Additionally, many external stakeholders such as health care networks, special interest groups/organizations, vendors, patients and families, the community, and third-party payors exert influence on health care organizations. Despite the diversity among these external factors, one common trend is the expectation that organizations base their health care practices and standards on sound evidence.

Internal factors can include organizational culture, values, and beliefs; practice environment (e.g., leadership, resource allocation, patient services, organizational mission and priorities, availability of technology, library support); equipment and supplies; staffing; and organizational standards. Enacting EBP within an organization requires

- A culture that believes EBP will lead to optimal patient outcomes

- Strong leadership support at all levels with the necessary resource allocation (human, technological, and financial) to sustain the process

- Clear expectations that incorporate EBP into standards and job descriptions

Knowledge and evaluation of the patient population, the health care organization, and the internal and external factors are essential for successful implementation and sustainability of EBP within an organization.

The JHNEBP Process: Practice Question, Evidence, and Translation

The 18-step JHNEBP process (Appendix D) occurs in 3 phases and can be simply described as Practice question, Evidence, and Translation (PET) (see Figure 3.3). The process begins with the identification of a practice problem, issue, or concern. This step is critically important because how the problem is posed drives the remaining steps in the process. Based on the problem statement, the *practice question* is developed and refined, and a search for *evidence* is conducted. The evidence is then appraised and synthesized. Based on this synthesis, a determination is made as to whether or not the evidence supports a change or improvement in practice. If the data supports a change, evidence *translation* begins and the practice change is planned, implemented, and evaluated. The final step in translation is dissemination of results to patients and families, staff, hospital stakeholders, and, if appropriate, the local and national community.

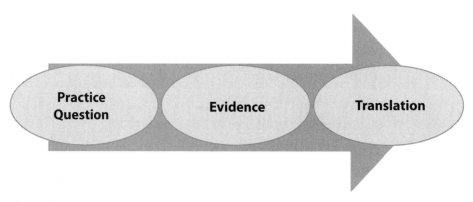

Figure 3.3   The JHNEBP PET Process: Practice Question, Evidence, and Translation
(© The Johns Hopkins Hospital/The Johns Hopkins University)

Practice Question

The first phase of the process (steps 1–5) includes forming a team and developing an answerable EBP question. An interprofessional team examines a practice concern, develops and refines an EBP question, and determines its scope. The Project Management Guide (see Appendix A) should be referred to frequently throughout the process to direct the team's work and gauge progress. The tool identifies the following steps.

Step 1: Recruit Interprofessional Team

The first step in the EBP process is to form an interprofessional team to examine a specific practice concern. It is important to recruit members for which the question holds relevance. When members are interested and invested in addressing a specific practice concern, they are generally more effective as a team. Bedside clinicians (or frontline staff) are key members because they likely have firsthand knowledge of the problem, its context, and impact. Other relevant stakeholders may include team members such as clinical specialists (nursing or pharmacy), members of committees or ancillary departments, physicians, dieticians, pharmacists, patients, and families. These may provide discipline-specific expertise or insights to create the most comprehensive view of the problem and, thus, the most relevant practice question. Keeping the group size to 6–8 members makes it easier to schedule meetings and helps to maximize participation.

Step 2: Develop and Refine the EBP Question

The next step is to develop and refine the clinical, educational, or administrative EBP question. It is essential that the team take the necessary time to carefully determine the actual problem (see Chapter 4). They need to identify the gap between the current state and the desired future state—in other words, between what the team sees and experiences and what they want to see and experience. The team should state the question in different ways and get feedback from nonmembers to see if any disagreement on the actual problem exists and if the question accurately reflects the problem. The time devoted to challenging assumptions about the problem, looking at it from multiple angles and obtaining feedback is always time well spent. Incorrectly identifying the problem results in wasted effort searching and appraising evidence that, in the end, does not provide the knowledge that allows the team to achieve the desired outcomes.

Additionally, keeping the question narrowly focused makes the search for evidence specific and manageable. For example, the question "What is the best way to stop the transmission of methicillin-resistant staphylococcus aureus (MRSA)?" is extremely broad and could encompass many interventions and all practice settings. In contrast, a more focused question is, "What are the best environmental strategies for preventing the spread of MRSA in adult critical-care units?" This narrows the question to environmental interventions, such as room cleaning; limits the age group to adults; and limits the practice setting to critical care. The PET process uses the PICO mnemonic (Sackett, Straus, Richardson, Rosenberg, & Haynes, 2000) to describe the four elements of a focused clinical question: (a) patient, population, or problem, (b) intervention, (c) comparison with other treatments, and (d) measurable outcomes (see Table 3.3).

Table 3.3   Application of PICO Elements

Patient, population, or problem	Team members determine the specific patient, population, or problem related to the patient/population under examination. Examples include age, sex, ethnicity, condition, disease, and setting.
Intervention	Team members identify the specific intervention or approach to be examined. Examples include interventions, education, self-care, and best practices.
Comparison with other interventions, if applicable	Team members identify what they are comparing the intervention to, for example, current practice or another intervention.
Outcomes	Team members identify expected outcomes based on the implementation of the intervention. The outcomes must include metrics that will be used to determine the effectiveness if a change in practice is implemented.

The Question Development Tool (see Appendix B) guides the team in defining the practice problem, examining current practice, identifying how and why the problem was selected, limiting the scope of the problem, and narrowing the EBP question using the PICO format. The tool also helps the team develop their search strategy by identifying the sources of evidence to be searched and possible search terms. It is important to recognize that the EBP team can go back and further refine the EBP question as more information becomes known as a result of the evidence search and review. Refer to Chapter 4 for more details regarding the development and refining of an EBP practice question.

Step 3: Define the Scope of the EBP Question and Identify Stakeholders

The EBP question may relate to the care of an individual patient, a specific population of patients, or the general patient population within the organization. Defining the scope of the problem assists the team in identifying the appropriate individuals and stakeholders who should be involved and kept informed during the EBP project. A stakeholder can be defined as an individual or organization that has an interest, personal or professional, in the topic under consideration (Agency for Healthcare Research and Quality, 2011). Stakeholders may include a variety of clinical and nonclinical staff, departmental and organizational leaders, patients and families, insurance payors, or policy makers. Identifying and including appropriate EBP team members and keeping key stakeholders informed can be instrumental to successful change. The team should consider whether the EBP question is specific to a unit, service, or department, or if it involves multiple departments. If the latter, a much broader group of individuals need to be recruited for the EBP team, with representatives from all areas involved. Key leadership in the affected departments should be kept up-to-date on the team's progress. If the problem affects multiple disciplines (e.g., nursing, medicine, pharmacy, respiratory therapy), each discipline should also be included.

Step 4: Determine Responsibility for Project Leadership

Identifying a leader for the EBP project is a key success factor. The leader facilitates the process and keeps it moving forward. The leader should be knowledgeable about evidence-based practice and have experience and a proven track record in leading interprofessional teams. It is also helpful if this individual knows the organizational structure and strategies for implementing change within the organization.

Step 5: Schedule Team Meetings

Setting up the first EBP team meeting can be a challenge and includes activities such as:

- Reserving a room with adequate space conducive to group discussion
- Asking team members to bring their calendars so that subsequent meetings can be scheduled
- Ensuring that a team member is assigned to record discussion points and group decisions
- Keeping track of important items (e.g., copies of the EBP tools, extra paper, dry erase board, and so on)
- Providing a place to keep project files
- Establishing a timeline for the process

Evidence

The second phase (steps 6–10) of the PET process deals with the search for, appraisal of, and synthesis of the best available evidence. Based on these results, the team makes recommendations regarding practice changes.

Step 6: Conduct Internal and External Search for Evidence

Team members determine the type of evidence to search for (see Chapter 5) and who is to conduct the search and then bring items back to the committee for review. Enlisting the help of a health information specialist (librarian) is critical. Such help saves time and ensures a comprehensive and relevant search. In addition to library resources, other sources of evidence include:

- Clinical practice guidelines
- Quality improvement data

- Position statements from professional organizations
- Opinions of internal and external experts
- Regulatory, safety, or risk management data
- Community standards
- Patient and staff surveys and satisfaction data

Step 7: Appraise the Level and Quality of Each Piece of Evidence

In this step, research and non-research evidence is appraised for level and quality. The Research Evidence Appraisal Tool (see Appendix E) and the Non-Research Evidence Appraisal Tool (see Appendix F) assist the team in this activity. Each tool includes a set of questions to determine the type, level, and quality of evidence. The PET process uses a five-level scale to determine the level of the evidence, with level I evidence as the highest and level V as the lowest (see Appendix C). Based on the questions provided on the tools, the quality of each piece of evidence is rated as *high, good,* or *low-major flaws.* The team reviews each piece of evidence and determines both the level and quality. Evidence with a quality rating of low-major flaws is discarded and not used in the process. The Individual Evidence Summary Tool (see Appendix G) tracks the team's appraisal of each piece of evidence, including the author, date, evidence type, sample, sample size, setting, and study findings that help to answer the EBP question, limitations, level, and quality. Chapters 6 and 7 provide a detailed discussion of evidence appraisal.

Step 8: Summarize the Individual Evidence

The team numerically sums the pieces (sources) of evidence that answer the practice question for each level (I–V) and records the totals on the Synthesis and Recommendations Tool (see Appendix H). The relevant findings that answer the EBP question for each level are then written in summary form next to the appropriate level.

Step 9: Synthesize Overall Strength and Quality of Evidence

Next, the team determines the overall quality for each level (I–V) and records it on the Synthesis and Recommendations Tool (see Appendix H). Through synthesis, the team makes a determination as to the overall strength and quality of the collected body of evidence, taking into consideration the: (a) level, (b) quantity, (c) consistency of findings across all pieces of evidence, and (d) applicability to the population and setting. The team can use the quality criteria for individual evidence appraisal as a guide for determining overall quality. Making decisions about the overall strength and quality is both an objective and subjective process. The EBP team should devote the necessary time to thoughtfully evaluate the body of evidence and come to agreement on the overall strength and quality. Refer to Chapters 6 and 7 and Appendix I for more information on evidence synthesis.

Step 10: Develop Recommendations for Change Based on Evidence Synthesis

Based on the overall appraisal and synthesis of the evidence, the team considers possible pathways to translate evidence into practice. A team has four common pathways to consider when developing a recommendation (Poe & White, 2010):

- Evidence may be compelling, with consistent results that support a practice change

- Evidence may be good, with consistent results that support a practice change

- Evidence may be good, but with conflicting results that may or may not support a practice change

- Evidence may be nonexistent or insufficient to support a practice change

Based on the selected translation pathway, the team then determines whether to make the recommended change or investigate further (see Table 3.4). The team lists its recommendations on the Synthesis and Recommendations Tool. The risks and benefits of making the change should be carefully considered. Initiating a change as a pilot study (with small sample size) to determine possible unanticipated adverse effects is strongly recommended.

Table 3.4   Translation Pathways for EBP Projects

	Evidence			
	Compelling, consistent	*Good, consistent*	*Good, but conflicting*	*Insufficient/ absent*
Make recommended change?	Yes	Consider pilot of change	No	No
Need for further investigation?	No	Yes, particularly for broad application	Yes, consider periodic review for new evidence or development of research study	Yes, consider periodic review for new evidence or development of research study
Risk-benefit analysis	Benefit clearly outweighs risk	Benefit may outweigh risk	Benefit may or may not outweigh risk	Insufficient information to make determination

Reprinted from Poe and White, 2010

Translation

In the third phase (steps 11–18) of the process, the EBP team determines if the changes to practice are feasible, appropriate, and a good fit given the target setting. If they are, the team creates an action plan, implements and evaluates the change, and communicates the results to appropriate individuals both internal and external to the organization.

Step 11: Determine Fit, Feasibility, and Appropriateness of Recommendation for Translation Pathway

The team communicates and obtains feedback from appropriate organizational leaders, bedside clinicians, and all other stakeholders affected by the practice recommendations to determine if the change is feasible, appropriate, and a good fit for the specific practice setting. They examine the risks and benefits of implementing the recommendations. They must also consider the resources available and the organization's readiness for change (Poe & White, 2010). Even with strong, high-quality evidence, EBP teams may find it difficult to implement practice changes in some cases. For example, an EBP team examined the best strategy for ensuring appropriate enteral tube placement after initial tube insertion. The evidence indicated that x-ray was the only 100% accurate method for identifying tube location. The EBP team recommended that a post-insertion x-ray be added to the enteral tube protocol. Despite presenting the evidence to clinical leadership and other organizational stakeholders, the recommendation was not accepted within the organization. Concerns were raised about the additional costs and adverse effects that may be incurred by patients (appropriateness). Other concerns related to delays in workflow and the availability of staff to perform the additional X-rays (feasibility). Risk management data showed a lack of documented incidents related to inappropriate enteral tube placement. As a result, after weighing the risks and benefits, the organization decided that making this change was not a good fit at that time.

Step 12: Create Action Plan

If the recommendations are a good fit for the organization, the team develops a plan to implement the recommended practice change. The plan may include:

- Development of (or change to) a protocol, guideline, critical pathway, system or process related to the EBP question

- Development of a detailed timeline assigning team members to the tasks needed to implement the change (including the evaluation process and reporting of results)

- Solicitation of feedback from organizational leaders, bedside clinicians, and other stakeholders

Essentially, the team must consider the *who, what, when, where, how,* and *why* when developing an action plan for the proposed change.

Step 13: Secure Support and Resources to Implement Action Plan

The team needs to give careful consideration to the human, material, or financial resources needed to implement the action plan. Obtaining support and working closely with departmental and organizational leaders can help to ensure the successful implementation of the EBP action plan.

Step 14: Implement Action Plan

When the team implements the action plan, they need to ensure that all affected staff and stakeholders receive verbal and written communication, as well as education about the practice change, implementation plan, and evaluation process. EBP team members should be available to answer any questions and troubleshoot problems that may arise during implementation.

Step 15: Evaluate Outcomes

Using the outcomes identified on the Question Development Tool (see Appendix B), the team evaluates the degree to which the outcomes were met. Although, of course, the team desires positive outcomes, unexpected outcomes often provide opportunities for learning, and the team should examine why these occurred. This examination may indicate the need to alter the practice change or the implementation process, followed by re-evaluation. The evaluation should also be incorporated into the organization's quality improvement process when ongoing measurement, evaluation, and reporting are indicated.

Step 16: Report Outcomes to Stakeholders

The team reports the results to appropriate organizational leaders, bedside clinicians, and all other stakeholders. Sharing the results, both favorable and unfavorable, helps disseminate new knowledge and generate additional practice or research questions. Valuable feedback obtained from stakeholders can overcome barriers to implementation or help develop strategies to improve unfavorable results.

Step 17: Identify Next Steps

EBP team members review the process and findings and consider if any lessons have emerged that should be shared or if additional steps need to be taken.

These lessons or steps may include a new question that has emerged from the process, the need to do more research on the topic, additional training that may be required, suggestions for new tools, the writing of an article on the process or outcome, or the preparation of an oral or a poster presentation at a professional conference. The team may identify other problems that have no evidence base and, therefore, require the development of a research protocol. For example, when the recommendation to perform a chest x-ray to validate initial enteral tube placement was not accepted (see the scenario discussed in step 11), the EBP team decided to design a research study to look at the use of colormetric carbon dioxide detectors to determine tube location.

Step 18: Disseminate Findings

This final step of the process is one that is often overlooked and requires strong organizational support. The results of the EBP project, at a minimum, need to be communicated to the organization. Depending on the scope of the EBP question and the outcome, consideration should be given to communicating findings external to the organization in appropriate professional journals or through presentations at professional conferences.

Summary

This chapter introduces the JHNEBP Model and the steps of the PET process. Nursing staff with varied educational preparation have successfully used this process with mentorship and organizational support. They have found it very rewarding both in understanding the basis for their current nursing interventions and incorporating changes into their practice based on evidence (Newhouse, Dearholt, Poe, Pugh, & White, 2005).

References

Agency for Healthcare Research and Quality. (2011). *Engaging stakeholders to identify and prioritize future research needs*. Retrieved from http://www.effectivehealthcare.ahrq.gov/index.cfm/search-for-guides-reviews-and-reports/?pageaction=displayproduct&productid=698

American Nurses Association. (2010). *Nursing: Scope and standards of practice*. Washington, DC: Author.

American Nurses Credentialing Center. (2011). *Announcing the model for ANCC's magnet recognition program.* Retrieved from http://www.nursecredentialing.org/Magnet/ProgramOverview/New-Magnet-Model.aspx

Institute of Medicine. (2003). *Health professions education: A bridge to quality.* Washington, DC: The National Academics Press.

Institute of Medicine. (2011). *The future of nursing: Leading change, advancing health.* Washington, DC: The National Academics Press.

Krahn, M., & Naglie, G. (2008). The next step in guideline development, incorporating patient preferences. *Journal of the American Medical Association, 300*(4), 436-438.

Melnyk, B. M., Fineout-Overholt, E., Stillwell, S. B., & Williamson, K. M. (2009). Igniting a spirit of inquiry: An essential foundation for evidence-based practice. *American Journal of Nursing, 109*(11), 49-52.

Newhouse, R., Dearholt, S., Poe, S., Pugh, L., & White, L. (2005). Evidence-based practice. *Journal of Nursing Administration, 35*(1), 35-40.

Oman, K. S., Duran, C., & Fink, R. (2008). Evidence-based policy and procedure. *Journal of Nursing Administration, 38*(1), 47-51.

Pape, T. M., & Richards, B. (2010). Stop "knowledge creep." *Nursing Management, 41*(2), 8-11.

Poe, S. S., & White, K. M. (2010). *Johns Hopkins nursing evidence-based practice: Implementation and translation.* Indianapolis, IN: Sigma Theta Tau International.

Porter-O'Grady, T. (1984). *Shared governance for nursing: A creative approach to professional accountability.* Rockville, Maryland: Aspen Systems Corporation.

Reigle, B. S., Stevens, K. R., Belcher, J. V., Huth, M. M., McGuire, E., Mals, D., & Volz, T. (2008). Evidence-based practice and the road to Magnet status. *Journal of Nursing Administration, 38* (2), 97-102.

Sackett, D. L., Straus, S. E., Richardson, W. S., Rosenberg, W., & Haynes, R. B. (2000). *Evidence-based medicine: How to practice and teach EBM.* Edinburgh: Churchill.

Wolf, G., Triolo, P., & Ponte, P. R. (2008). Magnet recognition program: The next generation. *Journal of Nursing Administration, 38*(4), 200-204.

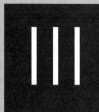

Practice Question, Evidence, Translation (PET)

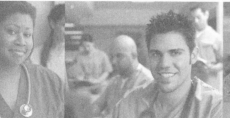
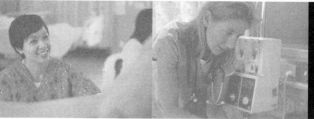

4

The Practice Question

Robin P. Newhouse, PhD, RN, NEA-BC, FAAN

Stephanie S. Poe, DNP, RN

Practice questions frequently arise from day-to-day problems encountered by clinicians, administrators, and nurse educators. Answers to these questions in the form of evidence are available in print or electronic media or through evidence summaries such as systematic reviews, integrative reviews, literature reviews, or guidelines. The objectives for this chapter, the first phase of the evidence-based practice (EBP) process, asking a practice question, are to:

- Identify the steps in forming an EBP team

- Illustrate how to define practice problems appropriate for an EBP approach

- Describe how to use the PICO framework to create an answerable EBP question

   The practice question phase of EBP research includes five operational steps. The first is to assemble an interprofessional team to examine a specific practice concern or problem. The team then works together to complete the other process steps: developing and refining the EBP question, defining the scope of the question, determining project leadership, and outlining the team's responsibilities. The Johns Hopkins Nursing Evidence-based Practice (JHNEBP) Question Development Tool (see Appendix B) facilitates this phase.

The Interprofessional EBP Team

Having appropriate interprofessional representation on the EBP team is critical to the team's success. Different team members should be included depending on the scope of the problem. For example, if the problem is post-operative hypothermia management, then representatives from anesthesia and surgery should be included. Anticipating how recommendations made by the team may be implemented and whose practice may be affected also helps determine which individuals or groups should be involved—either as team members or as stakeholders. The EBP team must consist of members who have expertise with the practice problem under consideration. Usually this means a team that includes nurses, physicians, and other professional staff who contribute significantly to care of the patient population selected. For example, if the question relates to best practices in the management of nausea for the patient undergoing chemotherapy, the team may consist of nurses, pharmacists, and oncologists. The number of members should be small enough to promote efficiency and large enough to provide content expertise—typically six to eight persons. Team members must agree to attend meetings, review and present evidence, participate in evidence synthesis, generate practice recommendations, and contribute to and support team decisions. Teams that have never before conducted an EBP project can benefit by recruiting an experienced mentor to help them through the process the first time.

After the team is assembled and ready to begin the EBP process, members select a team leader. This leader should be someone who can facilitate meetings, manage projects, articulate the team's recommendations, and influence implementation. The leader establishes a regular meeting schedule so members can reserve the time, which is sometimes the most challenging portion of planning the EBP project. Selecting a time and venue away from the demands of the clinical area and within a timeline realistic enough to complete the project is essential. Team members who work multiple shifts, various days, and in different roles can rarely agree on a time and date without as much as two months notice. Occasionally, teams with regularly scheduled meetings established for quality improvement, policy and procedure review, or other professional responsibility use a portion of this standard meeting time for the EBP project.

Some teams schedule a preliminary meeting to refine the practice question, then one or two eight-hour days to review evidence and make recommendations. Others have approached scheduling challenges by setting aside four-hour blocks of time monthly or five, two-hour meetings every other week. Scheduling meetings weekly if possible or every two weeks keeps the team moving forward. Delay between group meetings negatively affects the team's momentum.

Practice Problems

Interprofessional team members begin their task by defining the practice problem—a vital activity because all subsequent actions and decisions build on the clarity of the problem definition. The process often begins by seeking answers to practice concerns, such as

- Is there evidence that this treatment works?

- Does this practice help the patient?

- Why are we doing this practice, and should we be doing it this way?

- Is there a way to do this practice more efficiently or more cost-effectively?

The practice problem can emerge from multiple sources. Titler et al., in two classic publications (1994, 2001), identified problem-focused or knowledge-focused triggers as sources of problems. *Problem-focused triggers* are those identified by staff during routine monitoring of quality, risk, adverse event, financial, or benchmarking data. *Knowledge-focused triggers* are identified through reading published reports or learning new information at conferences or professional meetings. (See Table 4.1.)

Table 4.1   Sources of Evidence-Based Practice Problems

Triggers	Sources of Evidence
Problem-focused	Financial concerns
	Evidence for current practice questioned
	Quality concern (efficiency, effectiveness, timeliness, equity, patient-centeredness)
	Safety or risk management concerns
	Unsatisfactory patient, staff, or organizational outcomes
	Variations in practice compared with external organizations
	Variations in practice within the setting
Knowledge-focused	New sources of evidence
	Changes in standards or guidelines
	New philosophies of care
	New information provided by organizational standards committees

Problems may also be recurring or priority issues within an organization, or a practice that has questionable benefit. Clinical questions can seek to understand dissimilar outcomes in the same patient population. Why do some patients in the intensive care unit (ICU), for example, develop ventilator-associated pneumonia, whereas other ICU patients do not? There may be a difference in practice among nurses, nursing units, or peers outside of the organization. The potential for problems to generate practice questions is limitless, and EBP projects have the potential to result in improvements in health, organization of systems, or education. Problems that are important are those that can cause harm, result in an unsatisfactory experience, or cause high resource use. Important problems are worthy of consideration before beginning the EBP project so that time and effort are dedicated only to those questions with likely benefit.

The JHNEBP Question Development Tool (see Appendix B) can be used to create a practice question beginning with a clear statement of the problem or issue— the basis of any answerable EBP question. Time spent defining the problem clearly and concisely facilitates the construction of a strong EBP question. The goal is to convert the need for knowledge into an answerable question. Table 4.2 provides specific strategies for defining the EBP problem and gives an example of each.

Table 4.2   Strategies for Defining the EBP Problem

Strategies	Rationale
Phrase the problem statement in terms of the knowledge gap not the solution: *"Best strategies to manage patient pain immediate post discharge total knee replacement are not known,"* instead of *"Patients need a better pain management strategy for the immediate post-discharge period."*	Allows the team to see other, potentially more effective, solutions.
State the problem rather than symptoms of the problem: *"Forty percent of patients discharged post total knee replacement complain that they were not able to manage their pain,"* instead of *"Patients with total knee replacement were not satisfied after discharge."*	Allows the team to get to the true problem, its size and scope, without being sidetracked by outward signs that a problem exists.
Describe in precise terms the perceived gap between what one sees and what one would like to see: *"Patient satisfaction with pain management post discharge is 36% compared to a national benchmark of 85%."*	Allows the team to assess the current state and envision a future state in which broken things are fixed, risks are prevented, new evidence is accepted, and things that were missing are provided.
Examine the problem critically and make sure that the final statement defines the real problem: *"Do patients understand their pain management regimen?"* rather than, *"Are patients following the prescribed pain management regimen?"*	Gives the team time to gather information, observe, listen, and probe to ensure a true understanding of the problem.
Ask clarifying questions: *"When are these patients experiencing pain? What are the precipitating factors? How often are they taking their pain medications?"*	Question words such as "why" help the team get to the real problem.

Table 4.2   Strategies for Defining the EBP Problem (continued)

Strategies	Rationale
Refrain from blaming the problem on external forces or focusing attention on the wrong aspect of the problem.	Keeps the team focused on processes and systems as the team moves to define the EBP question.
Do not attribute blame, such as *"The patients are noncompliant with the prescribed pain medication therapy,"* or *"The nurses did not educate the patient properly about the importance of taking pain medications as prescribed."*	
State the problem in a different way: *"Forty percent of patients with post total knee replacement had low patient satisfaction scores related to pain management after discharge."*	Using different verbs can help to gain clarity.
Challenge assumptions. The team assumes the patient fills the pain medication prescription and is taking pain medication in the way that it was prescribed. *"Is this a correct assumption?"*	Helps the team to avoid conjecture and to question everyday things that are taken for granted.
Expand and contract the problem: *"Is dissatisfaction with post-discharge pain management part of a general dissatisfaction with the hospital stay as a whole?"* or *"Are there multiple reasons for dissatisfaction with post-discharge pain management, such as inability to pay for pain medications or fear of becoming dependent on pain medications?"*	Helps the team to understand if the problem is part of a larger problem or is made up of many smaller problems.
Assume multiple solutions: *"What are best practices for managing post-discharge pain in patients following total knee replacement?"* instead of *"What is the best practice for managing post-discharge pain in patients following total knee replacement?"*	Helps the team to identify more than one possible solution to determine best fit for the population of interest.

After the problem is identified, the team describes the current practice. This helps clarify specific processes that may be the source of the problem and establishes baseline data.

The team then defines the focus of the problem (clinical, educational, or administrative) and notes how the problem was identified. It is helpful to document such information on the Question Development Tool.

Determining the scope of the problem (individual, population, or system/organization) is the next charge for the team. Who is affected by the problem or concern? Where is it experienced? When does that problem surface? Defining the scope of the problem influences the selection of appropriate stakeholders who need to be informed or involved.

Evidence-based practice projects require time, availability of evidence, EBP skills, expert mentors, and leadership support. Consequently, the EBP model and process may not be practical for all questions. Choose questions that have a high return on quality processes, outcomes, and/or cost-efficiency. Before embarking on an EBP project and committing the time and resources necessary, consider the following questions: Would the practice changes resulting from this project improve clinical outcomes, unit processes, or patient or nurse satisfaction? Would they reduce the cost of care? Can potential practice changes be implemented given the current culture, practices, and organizational structure within the particular practice setting?

If the problem is important and a solution has the potential to improve the quality of care, then generating a focused question is the team's next step.

Practice Questions

Having agreed on the nature and scope of the practice problem, the EBP team develops an answerable question that addresses a clinical, administrative, or educational problem.

Background and Foreground Question

Two types of EBP questions exist—background and foreground (Sackett, Rosenberg, Gray, Haynes, & Richardson, 1996; Sackett, Straus, Richardson, Rosenberg, & Haynes, 2000). A *background question* is a general, best practice question that is broad and produces a wide range of evidence for review: "*What are the best nursing interventions to manage pain for patients with a history of substance abuse?*" This question would produce evidence related to pharmacology, alternative therapies, behavioral contracting, and biases in prescribing and administering pain medication. Evidence identified for background questions often provides the "state of the science" about a problem and can lead to a refined foreground question.

A *foreground question* is a focused question that includes specific comparisons: "*Is behavioral contracting or mutual goal setting more effective in improving the pain experience for patients with a history of substance abuse?*" Foreground questions produce a very refined, limited body of evidence specific to the EBP question.

When an EBP team is asking a background question, the evidence review can become complex. It is helpful to organize the EBP project by breaking down the components of the problem into the appropriate number of foreground questions. Create questions that relate to each of the components identified. For example, if the problem is high falls rates in older inpatients, the background question could be, "*What are the best practices in fall prevention for older patients?*" An appropriate foreground question could be, "*Which practice is more effective in reducing fall-related injury: bed alarms or hourly rounding?*"

Developing an Answerable EBP Question

The thoughtful development of a well-structured EBP question is important because the question drives the strategies used to search for evidence. Making the EBP question as specific as possible helps to identify and narrow search terms, which, in turn, reduces time spent searching for relevant evidence and increases the likelihood of finding it. Making the question as specific as possible focuses the EBP project and provides a sensitive evidence review that is specific to the problem and question. It also helps in clearly defining the target population, such as age, gender, ethnicity, diagnosis, and procedure, so that translation of the recommendations is planned appropriately. (Chapter 5 describes using keywords for evidence searches.)

A helpful format for constructing an answerable EBP question is Patient, Intervention, Comparison, and Outcome (PICO) (Richardson, Wilson, Nishikawa, & Hayward, 1995). PICO frames the problem clearly and facilitates the evidence search by identifying core keywords.

Patient, population, or problem

Describe the patient, population or problem succinctly. Include the type of patient or population and the setting. Consider attributes such as age, gender, and/or symptoms.

Intervention

The intervention can be a treatment; a clinical, educational, or administrative intervention; a process of care; nursing treatments; strategies for education; or assessment approaches.

Comparison with other intervention(s)

Determine if a comparison group exists. Will this intervention be compared to another? Not all questions have comparisons, particularly if you are asking a background question. A statement of current practice may be used as a comparison.

Outcomes that are measurable

Identify the outcomes of interest. Outcomes may include quality of life, improved treatment results, decreased rate of adverse events, improved patient safety, decreased cost, or improved patient satisfaction. The outcomes always include a metric for measuring results and the frequency for measuring and reporting results.

Table 4.3 provides an example using PICO to create a foreground question. The question is, "For adult surgical inpatients between the ages of 20 and 50 with a peripheral intravenous catheter, does the use of saline to flush the peripheral IV maintain IV patency and decrease phlebitis over 48 hours when compared to heparin flushes?"

Table 4.3   PICO Example of a Foreground Question

P—Patient, population, or problem	Adult surgical inpatients (patients), between the ages of 20 and 50 with a peripheral intravenous catheter (population)
I—Intervention	Use of saline flushes
C—Comparison	Use of heparin flushes for peripheral IV maintenance
O—Outcome	Improvements in IV patency over 48 hours, or a decrease in the incidence of phlebitis by 10%

The JHNEBP Question Development Tool provides a space for the team to record their initial EBP question. The question may be revised as the team conducts their evidence review. The tool also provides spaces for the team to brainstorm possible search terms and for evidence to be gathered.

Summary

This chapter introduces the multiple origins of practice problems appropriate for an EBP approach. It is essential to begin this first stage of the EBP project thoughtfully. The ultimate goal is a well-framed question developed by an appropriate interprofessional team who can complete the process successfully and efficiently.

References

Richardson, W. S., Wilson, M. C., Nishikawa, J., & Hayward, R. S. (1995). The well-built clinical question: A key to evidence-based decisions. *American College of Physicians, 123*(3), A12-A13.

Sackett, D. L., Straus, S. E., Richardson, W. S., Rosenberg, W., & Haynes, R. B. (2000). *Evidence-based medicine: How to practice and teach EBM*. Edinburgh: Churchill.

Sackett, K. L., Rosenberg, W. M., Gray, J. A., Haynes, R. B., & Richardson, W. S. (1996). Evidence based medicine: what it is and what it isn't. *British Medical Journal, 312*(7023), 71-72.

Titler, M. G., Kleiber, C., Steelman, V., Goode, C., Rankel, B., Barry-Walker, J., Small, S., & Buckwalter, K. (1994). Infusing research into practice to promote quality care. *Nursing Research, 43*(5), 307-313.

Titler, M. G., Kleiber, C., Steelman, V. J., Rakel, B. A., Budreau, G., Everett, ... Goode, C. J. (2001). The Iowa model of evidence-based practice to promote quality care. *Critical Care Nursing Clinics of North America, 13*(4), 497-509.

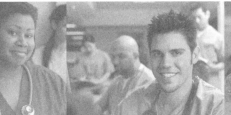
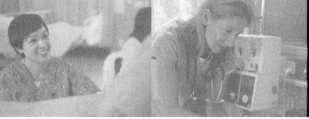

5

Searching for Evidence

Emily Munchel, RN, CPN
Stella Seal, MLS
Christina L. Wissinger, MS, MLIS

Developing information literacy skills requires knowledge of the nursing literature and an aptitude for locating and retrieving it. "Frequent review of bibliographic and full-text databases (i.e., any collection of records in an electronic form) that hold the latest studies reported in journals is the best, most current choice for finding relevant evidence to answer compelling clinical questions" (Fineout-Overholt, Nollan, Stephenson, & Sollenberger, 2010, p. 39). Studies have shown that positive changes in a nurse's information literacy skills and increased confidence in using those skills have a direct impact on appreciation and application of research, are vital for effective lifelong learning, and are a prerequisite to evidence-based practice (Shorten, Wallace, & Crookes, 2001).

Evidence can be collected from a variety of sources including the World Wide Web (www) and proprietary databases. The information explosion has made it difficult for health care workers, researchers, educators, and policy makers to process all the relevant literature available to them on a daily basis. Evidence-based clinical resources, however, have made searching for medical information much easier and faster than in years past. This chapter

- Describes key information formats
- Identifies steps in working with an answerable question
- Suggests information and evidence resources
- Provides tips for search strategies
- Suggests methods of evaluating search results

Key Information Formats

Nursing is awash with research data and resources in support of evidence-based nursing, which itself is continually evolving (Collins, Voth, DiCenso, & Guyatt, 2005). Evidence-based literature comes from many sources, and nurses need to keep them all in mind. The literature search is a vital component of the EBP process. If nurses search only a single resource, database, or journal, they will very likely miss important evidence. Through the search, nurses enrich their clinical practice and their experience in locating evidence important to the care they deliver.

Ideally, nurses looking for evidence to answer clinical or patient care questions can look first to the computerized patient record, which synthesizes patient information and provides search prompts based on that record (Straus, Richardson, Glasziou, & Haynes, 2011). Lacking such a system, however, nurses must look to other sources to find evidence in support of practice. Evidence falls into three main categories: *translation literature, evidence summaries,* and *primary evidence.*

Translation literature refers to evidence-based research findings that, after much research and analysis, have been translated into guidelines used in the clinical setting. It includes practice guidelines, protocols, standards, critical pathways, clinical innovations, evidence-based care centers, peer-reviewed journals, and bibliographic databases. Some sources of translation literature are the National Guideline Clearinghouse, the Best Practice Information Sheets of the Joanna Briggs

Institute, the Cumulative Index to Nursing and Allied Health Literature (CI-NAHL), and PubMed. (Information on accessing such resources is provided later in this chapter.)

Evidence summaries include systematic reviews, integrative reviews, meta-analysis, meta-synthesis, and evidence synthesis. These are summaries of the literature that identify, select, and critically appraise relevant research and use appropriate statistical or interpretive analysis to summarize the results of the studies. Evidence-based summaries can be found in library catalogs, online book collections, and online resources, such as PubMed, CINAHL, The Cochrane Library, the Joanna Briggs Institute, and the Database of Abstracts of Reviews of Effectiveness (DARE). For hospital administrators and case managers, Health Business Full Text is a source for quality improvement and financial information.

Primary evidence is data generally collected from direct patient or subject contact and includes hospital data, clinical trials, peer-reviewed research journals, conference reports and abstracts, and monographs, as well as summaries from data sets such as the Centers for Medicare & Medicaid Services Minimum Data Set. Databases where this information can be found include PubMed, CINAHL, Excerpta Medica Database (EMBASE), library catalogs, and institutional repositories. For hospital administrators, the Healthcare Cost and Utilization Project (HCUP) is a source for health statistics and information on hospital inpatient and emergency department use.

The Answerable Question

After a practice problem has been identified and converted into an answerable EBP question (see Chapter 4), the search for evidence begins with the following steps:

1. Identify the searchable keywords contained in the EBP question and list them on the Question Development Tool (see Appendix B). Include also any synonymous or related terms.

2. Identify the types of information needed to best answer the question and list the sources where such information can be found. What database(s) will provide the best information to answer the question?

3. Develop the search strategy.

4. Evaluate search results for validity, authority, and usefulness.

5. Revise the search strategy as needed.

6. Record the strategy specifics (terms used, limits placed, years searched) on the Question Development Tool and save the results.

EBP Search Examples

The first step in finding evidence is selecting searchable keywords from the answerable EBP question. The Question Development Tool facilitates this process by directing the team to identify the practice problem and, using the PICO components, to develop the search question.

For example, consider the following question: "What risk factors are associated with serious injury from falls in the adult acute care setting?" Some search terms to use may be *falls*, *risk factors*, *adults*, and *acute care settings*. Table 5.1 illustrates how the PICO format focuses these terms. However, additional terms such as *hospitals*, *injury*, *ambulatory care facilities*, and terms synonymous or linked to fall prevention could also be used.

Table 5.1   PICO Example: Risk Factors Associated with Injury from Falls

P (Population, setting):	Adults in acute care settings
I (Intervention):	Identification of fall injury risk factors
C (Comparison):	(Not applicable)
O (Outcome):	Decrease in serious injury from falls

Teams need to consider the full context surrounding the problem when thinking of search terms. As an example, *intervention* is a term used frequently in nursing; it comprises the full range of activities a nurse undertakes in the care of patients. Searching the literature for *nursing interventions*, however, is far too general and needs to be focused on specific interventions. In the preceding "Risk Factors Associated with Injury from Falls" example, possible interventions may include *medication, equipment,* and *floor coverings.* Table 5.2 shows the development of an answerable question for a specific EBP problem and the corresponding search strategy.

Table 5.2   Search Strategy for Distractions and Interruptions during Medication Administration

Problem

A hospital's quality improvement committee saw an increase in medication errors, and nurses indicated that distractions and interruptions were the largest contributing factor. Unit staff did not know what the best strategies were for controlling distractions and interruptions in their work environment during the medication administration process.

PICO

P (Population, setting):	Nurses on inpatient care units
I (Intervention):	Identification and control of distractions and interruptions in environment during medication administration
C (Comparison):	Current practice
O (Outcome):	Decrease in distractions and interruptions

Answerable Question

"What are the best practices to help nurses on inpatient units recognize and control interruptions and distractions during the medication administration process?"

Initial Search Terms	Related Search Terms
Hospital personnel	Nurses, physicians
Distractions	Health personnel
Medication errors	Attention, interruptions
Medication administration	

Selecting Information and Evidence Resources

After search terms have been selected, EBP teams can identify quality databases containing information on the topic. This section briefly reviews some of the unique features of core EBP databases in nursing and medicine.

CINAHL

The Cumulative Index to Nursing and Allied Health Literature (CINAHL) covers nursing, biomedicine, alternative or complementary medicine, and 17 allied health disciplines. CINAHL indexes more than 3,000 journals, contains more than 2.3 million records dating back to 1981, and has complete coverage of English-language nursing journals and publications from the National League for Nursing and the American Nurses Association (ANA). In addition, CINAHL contains health care books, nursing dissertations, selected conference proceedings, standards of practice, and book chapters. Full-text material within CINAHL includes more than 70 journals in addition to legal cases, clinical innovations, critical paths, drug records, research instruments, and clinical trials.

CINAHL also contains a controlled vocabulary called *CINAHL Subject Headings* that allows for more precise and accurate retrieval. Terms are searched using MH for Exact Subject Heading or MM for Exact Major Subject Heading. CINAHL also allows you to search using detailed limits to narrow results by publication type, age, gender, and language. The PICO on distractions could be searched using the CINAHL headings (MH "Distraction") AND (MH "Medication Errors") in combination with the keywords *distraction* and *medication errors*. The search strategy would look like this: ((MH "Distraction") OR distraction) AND ((MH "Medication Errors") OR "medication errors").

MEDLINE and PubMed

MEDLINE and PubMed are often used interchangeably; however, teams need to keep in mind that they are *not* the same. PubMed searches MEDLINE, but also searches articles that are not yet indexed in MEDLINE and articles that are included in PubMed Central.

MEDLINE, available free of charge through the National Library of Medicine's interface, PubMed, contains over 18 million references to journal articles in the life sciences with a concentration on biomedical research. One of MEDLINE's most notable features is an extensive, controlled vocabulary: *Medical Subject Headings* (MeSH). Each record in MEDLINE is reviewed by an indexer who is a specialist in a biomedical field. The indexer assigns an appropriate MeSH heading to every record, which allows for precise searching by eliminating irrelevant articles where a keyword may be casually mentioned. There is a saying in the library world: "Garbage in, garbage out." MeSH can eliminate "garbage," or irrelevant articles.

To search in PubMed using the PICO example for distractions during medication administration, one would use the MeSH for "Medication Errors" [MeSH]. MeSH has no term for "distractions," but *distraction*, as a keyword can be used. The related MeSH term of "Attention" [MeSH] could also be considered. The search strategy would look like this: ("Medication Errors"[MeSH] OR "medication errors"[All Fields]) AND ("Attention"[MeSH] OR distraction [All Fields]).

PubMed also contains *Clinical Queries*, which has pre-built evidence-based filters. Clinical Queries uses these filters to find relevant information on topics relating to one of five clinical study categories: therapy, diagnosis, etiology, prognosis, and clinical prediction guides. Clinical Queries also includes a search filter for systematic reviews. This filter combines search terms with a filter that limits results to systematic reviews, meta-analyses, reviews of clinical trials, evidence-based medicine, consensus development conferences, and guidelines.

The Cochrane Library

The Cochrane Library is a collection of databases that most notably includes the Cochrane Database of Systematic Reviews. Internationally recognized as the gold standard in evidence-based health care, Cochrane Reviews investigate the effects of interventions for prevention, treatment, and rehabilitation. They also assess the accuracy of a diagnostic test for a given condition in a specific patient group and setting. Over 4,500 Cochrane Reviews and as many as 2,000 protocols are currently available. Abstracts of reviews are available free of charge from the

Cochrane website; full reviews require a subscription. A medical librarian can identify the organization's access to this library.

Creating Search Strategies and Utilizing Free Resources

In the following section we will cover the necessary components used to create a solid search strategy. Databases are unique, so the components you select when creating a search strategy will vary; not every search strategy will utilize every component. The end of this section includes a list of free reliable resources with descriptions explaining the content available in each resource. Remember to check with your local medical library to see what additional resources may be available to you.

Key Components to Creating Search Strategies

After appropriate resources are identified to answer the question, the EBP team can now begin to create a search strategy. Keep in mind that this strategy needs to be adjusted for each database. Begin by breaking the question into concepts, selecting keywords and phrases that describe the concepts, and identifying appropriate, controlled vocabulary. Use *Boolean operators (AND, OR,* and *NOT)* to combine or exclude concepts. Remember to include spelling variations and limits where necessary. Note that the example search strategies for PubMed and CINAHL in the previous sections were created by combining the AND and OR Boolean operators.

Use OR to combine keywords and controlled vocabulary related to the same concept: ("Attention" [MeSH] OR distraction). Use AND to combine two separate concepts: ("Attention" [MeSH] OR distraction) AND ("Medication Errors" [MeSH] OR "medication errors").

Review the following steps to build a thorough search strategy:

1. Use controlled vocabularies when possible. Controlled vocabularies are specific terms used to identify concepts within an index or database. They

are important tools because they ensure consistency and reduce ambiguity where the same concept may have different names. Additionally, they often improve the accuracy of keyword searching by reducing irrelevant items in the retrieval list. Some well-known vocabularies are MeSH in MEDLINE (PubMed) and CINAHL Subject Headings in CINAHL. Nursing Interventions Classification (NIC) and Nursing Outcomes Classification (NOC) may be more familiar to those in the field of nursing.

2. Use the Boolean operators. Boolean operators are AND, OR, and NOT. Use OR to combine keywords and phrases with controlled vocabulary. Use AND to combine each of the concepts within your search. Use NOT to exclude keywords and phrases; use this operator with discretion to avoid excluding something relevant to the topic.

3. Use alternate spellings to create an exhaustive search. Remember, even within the English language you have spelling variations in American and British literature. In British literature, for example, *S*s often replace *Z*s and *OU*s often replace *O*s, to name a few—organisation versus organization, and behaviour versus behavior.

4. Use limits where appropriate. Most databases have extensive limits pages. PubMed and CINAHL allow you to limit by age, gender, species, date of publication, and language. The limit for publication types assist in selecting the highest levels of evidence: meta-analysis, practice guidelines, randomized controlled clinical trials, and controlled clinical trials.

Free Resources

Most databases require a paid subscription, but some are available free online. Table 5.3 lists quality resources available free on the Internet. Check the local medical or public library to see what is accessible. Medical librarians, knowledgeable about available resources and how each functions, can assist in the search for evidence and can provide invaluable personalized instruction. Never be afraid to ask for help! The only foolish question is the one unasked.

Table 5.3   Free Online Resources

Resource	Website
Joanna Briggs Institute (JBI)	www.joannabriggs.edu.au
Google Scholar	http://scholar.google.com/
National Guidelines Clearinghouse (NGC)	www.guideline.gov
NIH RePORTER: Research Portfolio Online Reporting Tool	http://report.nih.gov/
PubMed	www.ncbi.nlm.nih.gov/sites/entrez?db=PubMed
PubMed Central Homepage	www.pubmedcentral.nih.gov
Registry of Nursing Research: Virginia Henderson International Nursing Library	www.nursinglibrary.org/portal/main.aspx
The Cochrane Collaboration	www.cochrane.org
Turning Research into Practice (TRIP) Database: For Evidence-Based Medicine (EBM)	www.tripdatabase.com/index.html

The *National Guidelines Clearinghouse* (NGC) is a federal government resource that contains practice guidelines. NGC is available free of charge from the Agency for Healthcare Research and Quality (AHRQ); its mission is to provide a resource for objective, detailed information on clinical practice guidelines. The database includes summaries about the guidelines, links to full texts where available, and a guidelines comparison chart.

The *Joanna Briggs Institute* (JBI) is an international, not-for-profit, membership-based research and development organization. Part of the Faculty of Health Sciences at the University of Adelaide, South Australia, they collaborate internationally with over 70 entities. The Institute and its collaborating entities promote and support the synthesis, transfer, and utilization of evidence by identifying feasible, appropriate, meaningful, and effective practices to improve health care outcomes globally. JBI includes *Best Practice information sheets* that are produced specifically for health professionals and are based on evidence reported in systematic reviews.

The *Turning Research into Practice Database (TRIP)* is a clinical search tool designed to allow health professionals to rapidly identify the highest quality evidence for clinical practice. It searches hundreds of evidence-based medicine and nursing websites that contain synopses, clinical answers, textbook information, clinical calculators, systematic reviews, and guidelines.

The National Institutes of Health (NIH) *Research Portfolio Online Reporting Tool (RePORTER)* is a federal government database that lists federally funded biomedical research projects. NIH RePORTER replaced Computer Retrieval of Information on Scientific Projects (CRISP) in 2009. RePORTER retains all the search capabilities of CRISP and now includes additional query fields, hit lists that can be sorted and downloaded in Microsoft Excel, NIH funding for each project (expenditures), and publications and patents that have acknowledged support from each project (results).

The *Virginia Henderson International Nursing Library*, a service offered through the Honor Society of Nursing, Sigma Theta Tau International, offers nurses online access to reliable information that can be easily utilized and shared. The library's complimentary *Registry of Nursing Research* database allows searches of both study and conference abstracts. Primary investigator contact information is also available for requests of full-text versions of studies.

Google Scholar allows a broad search across many disciplines and sources for scholarly literature. It contains articles, theses, books and abstracts, and court opinions. Sources for content come from academic publishers, professional societies, online repositories, universities, and other websites. Google Scholar ranks documents by weighting the full text, publisher, and author(s), as well as how recently and frequently it has been cited in other scholarly literature.

The team can also gain valuable information by searching the table of contents of subject-related, peer-reviewed journals and by evaluating the reference list of books and articles cited in the works. All are valid ways to gather additional information.

Evaluating, Revising, and Storing Search Results

Whether EBP team members conduct a search individually or with the help of a medical librarian, it is the searcher's responsibility to evaluate the results for relevance and quality. Keep in mind that to answer the clinical question thoroughly, a team's search strategies may need several revisions, and they should allow adequate time for these alterations. A good way to eliminate lower quality literature in an initial review is to judge the resources using the following criteria (Johns Hopkins University—The Sheridan Libraries, 2010):

- *Who wrote it?* What is the author's affiliation, background, intent, or bias?

- *Who is the intended audience?* Is it intended for specialists, practitioners, the general public, or another targeted group?

- *What is the scope or coverage?* Is the resource meant to give a general overview, foundational introduction, detailed investigation, cutting-edge update, or some other level of detail?

- *Why was it written or published?* Is it meant to inform, explain, entertain, or persuade? Is it intended to be objective and neutral or controversial?

- *How current is it?* When was it published and last updated?

- *Where or by whom was it published?* Does this individual or group have a particular role or agenda? If relevant, what is the source of their funding?

- *How is the information presented?* Are sources or evidence cited? Are there bibliographies, footnotes, or other specific citations?

- *How accurate is it?* Is there an evidence trail? Are related sources cited to check with which to triangulate information or claims?

After a successful search strategy is created, teams or individuals should keep a record of the work. Often individuals research the same topic throughout their career so saving search strategies assists in updating work without duplication of effort. Most databases have a feature that allows saving a search within the database; however, it is always a good idea to keep multiple copies of searches. Microsoft Word documents or e-mails are a great way to keep a record of work.

PubMed is an example of a database that allows multiple searches to be saved. *My NCBI*, a companion piece to PubMed, permits users to create an account, save searches, set alerts, and customize preferences. Search results can also be saved by exporting them into a citation management software program such as *EndNote, RefWorks, Zotero,* and *Papers.* Though some citation management programs are free, others need to be purchased; some may be provided free by an organization. The function and capabilities of the various programs are similar.

After the citations are identified, the next step is to obtain the full text. If the full text is not available online, request the local library to obtain the information through their interlibrary loan service. This request may be free of charge if the local library is affiliated with a university or institute, but it may require a fee if the request for resources is made from a public library.

Summary

This chapter supports the multistep evidence-based practice model and uses the PICO as a guide for literature searches. An essential component of evidence-based practice, the literature search is important to any research and publication activity because it enables researchers to acquire a better understanding of the topic and an awareness of relevant literature. Information specialists, such as medical librarians, can help with complex search strategies and information retrieval.

Ideally researchers use an iterative search process: examining indexed databases, using keywords in searches, studying the resulting articles, and finally refining their searches for optimal retrieval. The use of keywords, controlled vocabulary, Boolean operators, and limits plays an important role in finding the most relevant material for the practice problem. Alerting services are effective in helping researchers keep up-to-date with a research topic. Exploring and selecting from the wide array of published information can be a time-consuming task, so plan carefully so that you can carry out this work effectively.

References

Collins, S., Voth, T., DiCenso, A., & Guyatt, G. (2005). Finding the evidence. In A. DiCenso, G. Guyatt, & D. K. Ciliska (Eds.), *Evidence-Based Nursing: A Guide to Clinical Practice*. St. Louis, MO: Elsevier Mosby.

Fineout-Overholt, E., Nollan, R., Stephenson, P., & Sollenberger, J. (2010). Finding relevant evidence. In B. M. Melnyk & E. Fineout-Overholt (Eds.), *Evidence-Based Practice in Nursing and Healthcare: A Guide to Best Practice* (2nd ed.) (pp. 39-69). Philadelphia, PA: Lippincott Williams & Wilkins.

Johns Hopkins University—The Sheridan Libraries. (2010). *Expository writing: The research process: Evaluating sources*. Retrieved from http://guides.library.jhu.edu/content.php?pid=24792&sid=179624

Shorten, A., Wallace, M. C., & Crookes, P. A. (2001). Developing information literacy: A key to evidence-based nursing. *International Nursing Review, 48*(2), 86-92.

Straus, S., Richardson, W. S., Glasziou, P., & Haynes, R. B. (2011). *Evidence-based medicine: How to practice and teach EBM* (4th ed.). Edinburgh: Churchill Livingstone.

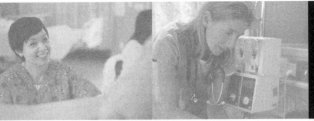

Evidence Appraisal: Research

Stephanie S. Poe, DNP, RN
Linda Costa, PhD, RN, NEA-BC

Most evidence rating schemes recognize that the strongest evidence accumulates from scientific evidence, also referred to as research. Within the broad realm of research, studies vary in terms of the level, quality, and strength of evidence they provide. The level of evidence is determined by the type of research design; the quality of evidence is determined by critical appraisal of study methods and execution; and the strength of evidence is determined through the synthesis of level and quality of evidence that leads to each practice recommendation (Jones, 2010). The current discussion of scientific evidence addresses the following types of research: summaries of multiple studies and individual research studies.

This chapter provides

- An overview of the various types of research evidence
- Tips for reading such evidence
- Information on appraising the strength and quality of research evidence

Publications That Report Scientific Evidence

Research evidence can be broadly grouped into reports of single research studies (experimental, quasi-experimental, non-experimental, and qualitative designs) and summaries of multiple research studies (systematic reviews with or without meta-analysis or meta-synthesis). The level of research evidence for single studies is determined by the study design. For summaries of multiple studies, the level of evidence is based on the collective designs of the studies included in the systematic review.

Most often, an evidence-based practice (EBP) team retrieves reports of primary research studies. *Primary* research comprises data that are collected to answer one or more research questions. Reviewers may also find *secondary* analyses that use data from primary studies to ask different questions. Evidence-based practice teams need to recognize and appraise each evidence type and the relative strength it provides. A working knowledge of the properties, strengths, and limitations of the various types of research studies enables the nurse to judge the relative quality of evidence.

Summaries of Multiple Studies

Published reports of research integrations, also referred to as systematic reviews, can be summaries of quantitative, qualitative, or both types of research. This section covers use of systematic reviews (with or without meta-analysis or meta-synthesis—defined later in this discussion) as tools to gather evidence. Notable efforts include The Cochrane Collaboration (2010a), an international nonprofit organization that produces and disseminates systematic reviews of health care interventions, and *Worldviews on Evidence-Based Nursing* (2011), a peer-reviewed journal developed by the Honor Society of Nursing, Sigma Theta Tau International. A less prominent, but growing effort to integrate and synthesize findings from qualitative research has been undertaken by the Cochrane Qualitative Research Methods Group. The *Cochrane Handbook for Systematic Reviews of Interventions* (Higgins & Green, 2011) includes a chapter providing guidance for using evidence from qualitative research to help explain, interpret, and apply the results of a Cochrane review.

Systematic Reviews

Systematic reviews summarize critically appraised research evidence (usually experimental and quasi-experimental studies) related to a specific question. Such reviews employ and document comprehensive search strategies and rigorous, transparent appraisal methods. Bias is minimized when a group of experts, rather than individuals, applies standardized methods to the review process.

A *systematic review* is interchangeable with an *evidence report*. The Agency for Healthcare Research and Quality (AHRQ) awards five-year contracts to North American institutions to serve as Evidence-based Practice Centers (EPCs). The EPCs review scientific literature on clinical, behavioral, organizational, and financing topics to produce evidence reports and technology assessments (AHRQ, 2011). Additionally, EPCs conduct research on systematic review methodology.

Sometimes systematic reviews are conducted as *integrative reviews*. Whereas classic systematic reviews include only experimental and quasi-experimental research, integrative reviews also include non-experimental studies and theoretical literature to arrive at full comprehension of the topic of interest (Tavares de Souza, Dias da Silva, & de Carvalho, 2010).

Systematic reviews often use *meta-analysis* or *meta-synthesis* to summarize the results of independent studies. When systematic reviews summarize the results of independent quantitative studies, they are referred to as meta-analysis. Meta-analysis provides a more precise estimate of the effects of health care interventions than those derived from individual studies included in the review (Higgins and Green, 2011). Through use of statistical methods, meta-analysis aids in understanding the consistency of evidence across studies.

In a systematic review with meta-analysis, statistical techniques are used to combine results from different studies to obtain a quantitative estimate of the overall effect of a particular intervention or variable on a defined outcome. Meta-analysis produces a stronger conclusion than can be provided by any individual study (The Cochrane Collaboration, 2010b).

When a systematic review summarizes the results of independent qualitative studies, they are referred to as a *meta-synthesis*. In a systematic review with a meta-synthesis, an attempt is made to combine results from a number of qualitative studies to arrive at a deeper understanding of the phenomenon under review. Meta-synthesis produces a broader interpretation than can be gained from a single qualitative study.

Systematic reviews differ from more traditional narrative literature reviews. Narrative reviews often contain references to research studies, but do not critically appraise, evaluate, and summarize the relative merits of the included studies. True systematic reviews address both the strengths and the limitations of each study included in the review. Readers should not differentiate between a systematic review and a narrative literature review based solely on the title of the article. Often the title will state that the article presents a literature review when, in fact, it is a systematic literature review. An example is "Failure to Rescue: A Literature Review" (Schmid, Hoffman, Happ, Wolf, & DeVita, 2007), which presents clear descriptions of methods of literature retrieval, as well as synthesis and appraisal of studies included in the review.

Evidence-based practice teams generally consider themselves lucky when they uncover well-executed systematic reviews that include summative research techniques that apply to the practice question of interest. Table 6.1 outlines the defining features of systematic reviews and reviews that include meta-analysis or meta-synthesis.

Table 6.1   Defining Features of Summative Research Techniques

Summative Evidence	Description	Defining Features
Systematic Review	Review of research evidence related to a specific clinical question	■ Employs comprehensive reproducible search strategies and rigorous appraisal methods ■ Can cover a range of research studies
Meta-analysis	Research technique that synthesizes and analyzes quantitative scientific evidence	■ Uses statistical procedures to pool results from independent primary studies ■ Usually includes experimental and/ or quasi-experimental studies ■ Estimates overall effect size of a specific intervention or variable on a defined outcome

Summative Evidence	Description	Defining Features
Meta-synthesis	Research technique that synthesizes and analyzes qualitative scientific evidence	<ul><li>Identification of key metaphors and concepts</li><li>Interprets and translates findings</li><li>Limited to qualitative studies</li></ul>

Meta-Analysis

A *meta-analysis* is a type of scientific evidence that quantitatively synthesizes and analyzes the findings of multiple primary studies that have addressed a similar research question (Polit & Beck, 2008). Meta-analysis uses "statistical techniques in a systematic review to integrate the results of included studies" (Moher, Liberati, Tetziaff, Altman, & the PRISMA Group, 2009, p. 1007). A meta-analysis can be based on individual patient data from primary studies that are similar enough to combine, or each primary study can serve as a unit of analysis. The strongest meta-analyses include only randomized controlled trials (RCTs). Meta-analyses that contain quasi-experimental studies rank below those that are restricted to RCTs.

A common metric called an *effect size* (ES), a measure of the strength of a relationship between two variables, is developed for each of the primary studies. A positive effect size indicates a positive relationship (as one variable increases, the second variable increases); a negative effect size indicates a negative relationship (as one variable increases or decreases, the second variable goes in the opposite direction). By combining results across a number of smaller studies, the researcher can increase the power, or the probability, of detecting a true relationship between the intervention and the outcomes of the intervention (Polit & Beck, 2008). When combining studies for meta-analysis, the researcher can statistically analyze only those independent variables and outcomes (dependent variables) that the studies have in common.

An *overall summary statistic* combines and averages effect sizes across studies. An investigator should describe the method that determined the effect size and should help the reader interpret the statistic. Cohen's (1988) methodology for determining effect sizes includes the following strength of correlation ratings:

trivial (ES = 0.01–0.09), low to moderate (0.10–0.29), moderate to substantial (0.30–0.49), substantial to very strong (0.50–0.69), very strong (0.70–0.89), and almost perfect (0.90–0.99).

> ### Example: Meta-Analysis
> London-based nurse researchers (Wu, Forbes, Griffiths, Milligan, & While, 2010) conducted a systematic review of randomized controlled trials to examine the effect of telephone follow-up on glycemic control. They applied statistics to the pooled results of five independent but similar (heterogeneous) studies that had sufficient data to include in a meta-analysis. The independent variable was telephone follow-up and the dependent variable (outcome) examined was HbA(1c) levels.

Meta-Synthesis

In contrast to numbers-based quantitative research, qualitative research is text-based. Qualitative researchers collect rich narrative materials; integration of these data results in a grand narrative or interpretative translation (Polit & Beck, 2008). Meta-synthesis is thought of as the qualitative counterpart to meta-analysis, but involves interpreting rather than aggregating data or producing a summary statistic (Beck, 2009a). Both use rigorous scientific techniques.

A number of different types of meta-synthesis methods exist. The most commonly used method is *meta-ethnography* with compares metaphors (concepts, themes, and phrases) included in individual qualitative studies and synthesizes these translations into an interpretation that is expressed visually through the written work, plays, art, or music (Beck, 2009a). Originating in the field of education as an alternative to meta-analysis (Noblit & Hare, 1988, p. 5), meta-ethnography answers the question of "how to 'put together' written interpretive accounts" and includes qualitative research using diverse methodological approaches (Barnett-Page & Thomas, 2009). Other meta-synthesis methods include *grounded theory, thematic synthesis, textual narrative synthesis, meta-study, meta-narrative,* and *ecological triangulation* (Barnett-Page & Thomas, 2009). For nurses who lack experience and expertise in critiquing qualitative studies, meta-syntheses are very helpful because they aid not only in assessing the rigor of individual studies, but also in interpreting findings.

> **Example: Meta-Synthesis**
>
> Schmied and colleagues (2011) conducted a qualitative meta-synthesis examining women's perceptions and experiences of breastfeeding support. They synthesized 31 studies that either were qualitative or had qualitative elements, summarizing categories and themes that emerged from the synthesis to illuminate the components of support that women actually deem to be "supportive."

Individual Research Studies

The EBP team begins its evidence search in hopes of finding the highest level of scientific evidence available on the topic of interest. Table 6.2 outlines the distinctive features of the various types of research evidence the team may uncover.

Table 6.2   Distinctive Features of Research Studies

Design	Distinctive Features	Examples
Experimental	■ An intervention ■ Control group ■ Random assignment to the intervention or control group ■ Manipulation of independent variable	■ Randomized controlled trial
Quasi-experimental	■ An intervention ■ May have a control group ■ Lacks random assignment to the intervention or control group ■ Some manipulation of independent variable	■ Non-equivalent control (comparison) group: post-test only or pre-test–post-test ■ One group: post-test only or pre-test–post-test ■ Time series ■ Untreated control, repeated measures ■ Repeated treatment where subjects serve as their own controls ■ Crossover design

Table 6.2   Distinctive Features of Research Studies (continued)

Design	Distinctive Features	Examples
Non-experimental (quantitative)	■ May have an intervention ■ No random assignment to a group ■ No control group ■ No manipulation of independent variables	■ Descriptive ■ Predictive ■ Explanatory ■ Time-dimensional ■ Case study
Qualitative	■ No randomization ■ No manipulation of independent variables ■ Little control of the natural environment	■ Historical research ■ Grounded theory ■ Ethnographic ■ Phenomenological-hermeneutic ■ Narrative analysis

Experimental Studies

Experimental studies, or randomized controlled trials (RCTs), use the traditional scientific method. The investigator obtains verifiable, objective, research-based knowledge by observing or measuring in a manner such that resulting evidence is reproducible. Types of experimental designs that an EBP team may encounter include pre-test–post-test control group (the original, most widely used experimental design); post-test only; factorial, randomized block; and crossover/repeated measures (Polit & Beck, 2008).

A true experimental study has three distinctive features: *randomization, control,* and *manipulation. Randomization* occurs when the researcher assigns subjects to a control or experimental group on a random basis, similar to the roll of dice. This ensures that each potential subject who meets inclusion criteria has the same probability of selection for the experiment. That is, people in the experimental group and in the control group generally will be identical, except for the introduction of the experimental intervention or treatment. This is important because subjects who take part in an experiment serve as representatives of the population the researcher feels may possibly benefit in the future from the intervention or treatment.

Manipulation is the researcher doing something to at least some of the subjects. An experimental intervention is applied to some subjects (the *experimental group*) and withheld from others (the *control group*) in an effort to influence some aspect of their health and well-being. The aspect that the researcher is trying to influence is the *dependent variable* (e.g., the experience of low back pain). The experimental intervention is the *independent variable*, or the action the researcher is going to take (e.g., application of low-level heat therapy) to try to change the dependent variable.

Control usually refers to the introduction of a control or comparison group, such as a group of subjects to which the experimental intervention is *not* applied. The goal is to compare the effect of no intervention on the dependent variable in the control group against the effect of the experimental intervention on the dependent variable in the experimental group. Use of a placebo is recommended whenever possible as some subjects may react to the placebo itself; this is termed the *placebo effect*.

Example: Experimental Randomized Controlled Trial

Jones, Duffy, and Flanagan (2011) reported on an experimental study testing the efficacy of a nurse-coached intervention in arthroscopy patients at a large, northeastern academic medical center. In this study, the researchers randomly assigned (*randomization*) subjects to a usual practice (*control*) group or to a nurse-coached telephone intervention (*manipulation*) group.

Quasi-Experimental Studies

Quasi-experimental designs are similar to experimental designs in that they try to show that an intervention causes a particular outcome. These designs are used when it is not practical, ethical, or possible to randomly assign subjects to experimental and control groups. They involve some degree of investigator control and manipulation of an independent variable. However, they lack randomization, the key ingredient of experimental studies. Because randomization is absent, the researcher makes some effort to compensate for the lack of random assignment, such as using multiple groups or multiple waves of measurement (Trochim, 2006). For example, an investigator can randomly assign the intervention to one of two groups, e.g., two medical units, with one serving as the intervention and one serving as the control. The investigator cannot randomly assign participants to the units, so this is not considered a randomized experiment. The unknown in this case is how participants are assigned to units and if it is unbiased and similar to chance (Gliner, Morgan, & Leech, 2009).

In cases where a particular intervention is effective, withholding that intervention would be unethical. In the same vein, it would not be practical to perform a study that requires more human, financial, and material resources than are available. At times neither patients nor geographical locations can be randomized. Consider the investigator who wants to study the effect of bed-exit alarms on patient falls. It would not be easy to randomize the use of bed-exit alarms to individual patient rooms or to individual patients because nursing staff likely would not agree to deactivate bed-exit alarms on at-risk patients whose beds are equipped with this safety feature. Quasi-experimental designs that an EBP team may uncover during the course of its search include non-equivalent control (comparison) group post-test only and non-equivalent control (comparison) group pre-test–post-test. The term *non-equivalent* means that not only is assignment non-random, but the researcher does not control assignment to groups. Hence, groups may be different on important variables such as health status or demographics, and group differences may affect outcomes. Other quasi-experimental designs include one group post-test only, one group pre-test–post-test, time series, untreated control with repeated measures, repeated treatment where subjects serve as their own controls, and crossover design (where the same subjects at different times receive both the experimental and the control intervention).

Examples: Quasi-Experimental Studies

Ceber, Turk, and Ciceklioglu (2010) conducted a study using a post-test only, control group design to examine the effect of an educational program on breast cancer-related knowledge, beliefs, and behaviors in nurses and midwives. This study is quasi-experimental rather than purely experimental because, although it included both an education program as the intervention (*manipulation*) and no education program for the control group (*control*), the subjects were not randomized to each group.

Yoo, Kim, Hur, and Kim (2011) employed a non-equivalent control group pre-test–post-test design to examine the effects of an animation distraction intervention on pain response of preschoolers during venipuncture. Again, this study included a distraction as the intervention (*manipulation*) and no distraction for the control (*control*) group, but subjects were recruited from a convenience sample (*non-random*).

Non-Experimental Studies

When reviewing evidence related to health care questions, particularly inquiries of interest to nursing, EBP teams are going to find that most published studies are non-experimental, or observational, in design. Non-experimental research involves the study of naturally occurring phenomena (groups, treatments, and individuals). These studies may or may not introduce an intervention. Subjects are not randomly assigned to different groups, variables are not manipulated, and the investigator is not always able to control aspects of the environment.

Quantitative non-experimental studies can be classified by research purpose and by time dimension (Belli, 2009). Three categories classified by purpose, or intent, are *descriptive, predictive,* and *explanatory.* Categories classified by time are *prospective, longitudinal,* and *retrospective.*

Descriptive Designs

The intent of purely descriptive designs, as the name implies, is to *describe* characteristics of phenomena. Basic questions asked in descriptive research are, "What are the quantifiable values of particular variables for a given set of subjects? How prevalent is a phenomenon?" Variables are not manipulated, and no attempt is made to determine that a particular intervention or characteristic causes a specific occurrence to happen. The investigators seek to provide the *who, what, where, when,* and *how* of particular persons, places, or things. An attempt is made to describe the answers to these questions in precisely measured terms. Statistical analysis is generally limited to frequencies and averages. Common types of descriptive designs include *univariate descriptive* (which often use exploratory or survey methods), *descriptive comparative, descriptive correlational,* and *epidemiologic descriptive* studies (prevalence and incidence).

Univariate descriptive studies, which often use exploratory or survey designs, aim to describe the frequency of a behavior or occurrence. Univariate descriptive studies are "not necessarily focused on only one variable … There are multiple variables … but the primary purpose is to describe the status of each and not to relate them to one another" (Polit & Beck, 2008). Exploratory and survey designs are common in nursing and health care. When little knowledge about the phenomenon of interest exists, these designs offer the greatest degree of flex-ibility. Though new information is learned, the direction of the exploration may change. With exploratory designs, the investigator does not know enough about a phenomenon to identify variables of interest completely. Variables are observed as they happen; no researcher is in control. When investigators know enough about a particular phenomenon and can identify specific variables of interest, a descriptive survey design more fully describes the phenomenon. Questionnaire (survey) or interview techniques assess the variables of interest.

> **Example: Non-Experimental Descriptive Survey Design**
>
> Palumbo, Marth, and Rambour (2011) used data from four biennial surveys to describe the demographic, educational, employment, job satisfaction, intent to leave, and practice-setting characteristics of the advanced practice nurse work-force in their state. There was no intervention, researcher control, or randomiza-tion; the intent was merely to describe existing characteristics.

Descriptive comparative designs look at and describe differences in variables between or among two or more groups. No attempt is made to determine causal-ity. Generally, descriptive statistics, such as frequency distributions and measures of central tendency (mean, median, and mode), are used to summarize these dif-ferences.

> **Example: Non-Experimental Descriptive Comparative Design**
>
> Hill (2011) employed a cross-sectional descriptive comparative design to exam-ine differences among work satisfaction, intent to stay, and financial knowledge of income-related retirement consequences between two groups (clinical bedside nurses and advance practice nurses). Researchers administered a series of ques-tionnaires (surveys) to a convenience sample (*non-random*) and described differ-ences in responses between the two groups.

Descriptive correlational designs seek to describe relationships among variables. Again no attempt is made to understand causal relationships. The in-vestigator gathers information on at least two variables, conducts a statistical correlation analysis between the two variables of interest to obtain a *correlation coefficient*—a number ranging from –1 to 1. The correlation coefficient tells the *direction* of the association between the two variables. If the correlation coefficient is between 0 and 1, the correlation is positive, meaning that as one variable of interest increases, so does the second variable. A negative correlation is depicted by correlation coefficients between –1 and 0, meaning that as one variable increases, the other variable decreases. The correlation coefficient also tells the reader the strength or *magnitude* of the correlation—that is, the closer this coefficient is to 1 (if positive) or –1 (if negative), the stronger the association between the two variables.

Example: Non-Experimental Descriptive Correlational Design

Researchers sought to examine emotional intelligence and nursing performance among nursing students (Beauvais, Brady, O'Shea, & Griffin, 2011). The researchers used Pearson's *r* Product Moment Correlation to describe the relationship of students' performance on an ability-based measure of emotional intelligence and on a six-dimension nursing performance measure. They found that professional development had a moderate correlation (*r* = 0.35) with total emotional intelligence score, whereas teaching and collaboration, planning and evaluation, and interpersonal relationships and communication had weak relationships (*r* = 0.22, 0.23, and 0.26, respectively).

Prevalence and incidence studies are descriptive designs frequently used by epidemiological researchers (Polit & Beck, 2008). The aim of prevalence studies is to determine the proportion of a population that has a particular condition at a specific point in time (known as prevalence or point prevalence). This provides researchers with a useful metric to better understand the burden of a specific disease in the community. Incidence studies seek to determine the frequency of new case (or incidence rate) and are useful in understanding risk for disease development.

Example: Non-Experimental Epidemiological Descriptive Designs

An interdisciplinary research team (Dybitz, Thompson, Molotsky, & Stuart, 2011) studied the prevalence of diabetes and the burden of comorbid conditions in elderly nursing home residents. Prevalence of diabetes was determined by laboratory values recorded in the medical record over a 12-month period, documented medical chart diagnosis of diabetes, and evidence of medications prescribed for diabetes in a prescription claims database. They found a diabetes prevalence of 32.8% of residents from a national sample of 250 skilled nursing facilities and characterized the disease burden of diabetes in these settings.

Roberts (2010) conducted electronic chart reviews of hospitalized children in a midsized urban hospital over a two-week period to determine the incidence of parental/guardian absence in the previous 24 hours. The researchers were interested in understanding the risk for unaccompanied pediatric patients in a culture that promotes patient-family centered care.

Predictive Designs

Predictive designs seek to *predict* relationships. Basic questions asked in predictive research are, "If phenomenon X occurs, will phenomenon Y follow? If we introduce an intervention, will a particular outcome follow?" Predictive designs range from simple predictive correlational studies that look at whether a single variable predicts a particular outcome to more complex predictive designs that use multiple or logistic regression to examine whether several variables predict a particular outcome.

Example: Non-Experimental Predictive Correlational Design

Mazanec, Daly, Douglas, and Musil (2011) used a predictive correlational design to examine the role of cognitive appraisal in predicting post-radiation treatment psychological adjustment in women with various forms of cancer. The research team prospectively examined the relationship between cognitive appraisal and the outcome variable (psychological adjustment).

Explanatory Designs

Explanatory designs seek to understand the foundation for and relationships among specific natural phenomena, and are often linked to theories (Polit & Beck, 2008). Basic questions for explanatory research are, "What does a particular phenomenon look like? Does a particular theory explain the phenomenon of interest?"

> **Example: Non-Experimental Explanatory Design**
>
> A population health research team (Chazelle et al., 2011) sought to explain social inequalities in mental health disorders. They used a descriptive explanatory design to examine the contribution of various factors to the association of educational level, major depression, and generalized anxiety disorder in the Irish population. They found that lack of private health insurance, no car, housing tenure, insufficient food budget, and unemployment in men made the highest contribution in explaining the association between education and both mental disorders.

Time-Dimensional Designs

Time-dimensional designs answer questions such as, "Were the data collected at a single point in time, across some time period, or did data already exist?" An EBP team should understand the concepts of retrospective, prospective, and longitudinal with respect to examining a phenomenon over time. In *retrospective* studies, the investigator looks at proposed causes and the effects that have already happened to learn from the past. In contrast, *prospective* studies examine causes that may have occurred in the past and then look forward in time to observe the presumed effects. *Longitudinal* studies look at changes in the same subjects over time. The basic question asked in longitudinal (present) and prospective (future) research is, "What are the differences in a variable or variables over time, going from the present to the future?" The basic question in retrospective studies is, "What differences in a variable or variables existed in the past that may explain present differences in these variables?"

Three common types of descriptive or observational studies that have a time component are *case-control*, *cohort*, and *cross-sectional*. Because unfamiliar terminology can divert the reviewer's attention from review of a study, an understanding of these terms should minimize confusion.

Case-control studies are used in epidemiologic research and examine possible relationships between exposure and disease occurrence. "The hallmark of the case-control study is that it begins with people with the disease (cases) and compares them to people without the disease (controls)" (Gordis, 2009, p. 179). The basic question asked in case-control studies is, "Is there a relationship between being exposed to particular phenomena and contracting a specific disease?"

Case-control studies compare the proportion of cases that have a particular condition or outcome with the proportion of cases that do not have the condition or outcome (Lu, 2009). This proportion is expressed as an *odds ratio*, which is a way of comparing whether the probability of a certain condition or outcome occurring is the same as the probability of the condition or outcome not occurring. An illustration of a case-control study (Figure 6.1) considers body mass index (BMI) as a determinant of obesity in the population of interest:

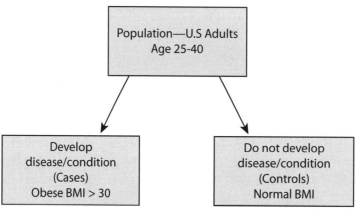

Figure 6.1   Illustration of a Case-Control Study

Example: Non-Experimental Descriptive Case-Control Design

A team of interdisciplinary researchers used a case-control design to look at risk factors for hospital-acquired poor glycemic control (McHugh, Shang, Sloane, & Aiken, 2011). This study compared hospital and patient characteristics in subjects (cases) who were identified as developing manifestations of poor glycemic control not present on admission with these same characteristics in a matched control group of patients (controls) who did not develop poor glycemic control. Odds ratios were calculated to estimate the effect of particular characteristics on development of poor glycemic control.

Cohort studies look at a particular subset of a population from which different samples are taken at various points in time. These types of observational studies can be retrospective, in which both the exposure and the outcome of interest has already occurred, or prospective, in which the patients who have been exposed to the condition of interest are observed to determine the occurrence of the outcome of interest (Lu, 2009). Cohort studies that are prospective may require a long-term follow-up period until the outcome event has occurred (Gordis, 2009). The risk factor of smoking in the population is used to illustrate a prospective cohort study (Figure 6.2):

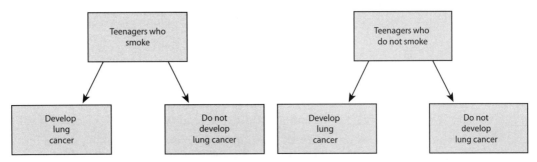

Figure 6.2   Illustration of a Prospective Cohort Study

Example: Non-Experimental Descriptive Cohort Design

A group of interdisciplinary researchers used a prospective cohort research design to examine the development of post partum depression in women who delivered single live infants at term (Sword et al., 2011). In this study, the defined population (cohort) was women greater than 15 years of age who delivered single live infants at term. They were not randomly assigned to a delivery mode, but were followed to see what delivery mode occurred naturally (exposure). Then each delivery group was followed to see if they developed post-partum depression within six weeks of delivery (outcome of interest).

Cross-sectional studies involve the collection of data at one particular point in time. These studies collect a representative sample and classify by outcome and risk factor simultaneously. The basic question asked in cross-sectional research is, "What are the characteristics of a population at a single point in time?" In epidemiology, the researcher starts with a defined population and gathers data on the presence or absence of exposure and the presence or absence of disease for each individual at a particular point in time. Prevalence studies employ epidemiological cross-sectional designs. In other types of studies using a cross-sectional design, the researcher looks at variables in a population at a single point in time.

> **Example: Non-Experimental Descriptive Cross-Sectional Design**
>
> Occupational health researchers used a cross-sectional observational study to examine the contribution of work activity, floor surface factors, demographic, and medical characteristics to the prevalence of hip disorders in assembly plant workers (Werner, Gell, Hartigan, Wiggermann, & Keyserling, 2011). In this study, the defined population was assembly plant workers. Investigators gathered data on exposure to work activity, floor surfaces, and medical characteristics to determine the prevalence of hip disorders. Data were gathered at a single point in time.

Qualitative Designs

Qualitative designs represent a unique category of descriptive research in that they challenge the traditional scientific worldview. Qualitative nurse researchers summarize and interpret data from a naturalistic worldview, which allows for multiple interpretations of reality, to develop insights into the meaning of the life experiences of patients (Beck, 2009b). Examples of qualitative designs include *historical research, grounded theory, ethnographic, phenomenological-hermeneutic,* and *narrative analysis.*

Historical designs use narrative description or analysis of events that occurred in the remote or recent past to discover facts and relationships (Polit & Beck, 2008). These data are categorized as primary (firsthand) or secondary (secondhand) sources and can include interviews, written documents, diaries, letters, and pictures (Beck, 2009b). The preference is to use primary sources whenever possible.

> **Example: Qualitative Historical Research Design**
>
> Ruffin (2011) examined massage in training school curricula from 1860–1945. By searching primary textbooks, journals, nursing curriculum guidelines, and archival collections, this researcher traced the roots of massage to refocus attention on mind-body healing and the importance of touch.

Grounded theory designs seek to examine the basic social and psychological problems/concerns that characterize real-world phenomena and to identify the process used to resolve these problems/concerns (Polit & Beck, 2008). In this type of qualitative research design, the researcher simultaneously collects and analyzes data to generate concepts and integrate these concepts into a data-grounded theory (Beck, 2009a). Data analysis is done through coding.

Example: Qualitative Grounded Theory Design

Allen (2011) used a grounded theory qualitative design to explore women's responses to intimate partner violence. Narrative interviews that encouraged each subject to tell her story were transcribed into a vast amount of data, to which grounded theory tools, including coding, were applied. This resulted in the emergence of a theory that the researchers used to better understand the practices and concerns of abused women as they move through their life experiences.

Ethnography describes and analyzes characteristics of the ways of life of cultures or subcultures and is of growing interest to nurses who seek to provide culturally competent care. The researcher is required to gain entry into the culture being studied, observing the behaviors of people in the culture while simultaneously participating in the activities (Beck, 2009b). Researchers immerse themselves in the culture of interest and keep extensive field notes, which are categorized and analyzed to discover major themes.

Example: Qualitative Ethnography Design

Knowles (2011) employed ethnography as one component of her qualitative study examining resilience among Japanese atomic bomb survivors. The researcher entered into a partnership and training experience with a binational Japan-United States scientific organization that studies health effects of atomic bomb radiation for peaceful aims. Ethnography was used to carefully explore artifacts provided by participants (such as photographs, written narratives, or diaries) and to incorporate these aspects into data analysis.

Hermeneutic phenomenology, developed by van Manen (1997), is both a descriptive (phenomenological) methodology in that it lets a phenomenon speak for itself and an interpretive (hermeneutic) methodology in that it claims that all phenomena can be interpreted. This qualitative research method examines an experience as people live it rather than as they conceptualize it. The researcher reflects on essential themes that characterize the experience through coding and categorization, writing, and rewriting (Chong & Poon, 2011).

> **Example: Qualitative Hermeneutic Phenomenology Design**
>
> Fouquier (2011) employed hermeneutic phenomenology in her qualitative study of the concept of motherhood among three generations of African-American women. This methodology allowed the researcher to interpret the human experience using language and knowledge of African-American culture and traditions and to develop a rich interpretation of patterns and relational themes related to the topic of interest.

Because qualitative and quantitative research designs are complementary, many studies use a combination of both. Though quantitative and qualitative studies both use very systematic processes, they have distinct differences in their worldviews.

- Quantitative studies are objective; they test theory (deductive), involve the use of numbers, and produce findings that are meant to be generalizable.

- Qualitative studies are subjective; they gain knowledge through the process of induction, involve use of words, and produce findings that are not meant to be generalizable.

After the EBP team has determined the level of research evidence based on study design, team members need to assess the quality of the evidence. To best assess quality, the team needs to understand how to interpret research evidence.

Interpreting Primary Research Evidence

To consider statistical information presented in reports of research evidence effectively, an EBP team needs a basic understanding of a study's *validity*, *reliability*, and *precision*. Validity is the extent to which the research measures what it intended to measure and how well the findings approximate the truthfulness of the subject of interest. Reliability refers to the consistency or repeatability of measurement. Precision has to do with how to interpret statistical measures of central tendency and clinical and statistical significance.

Measures of Validity

Measures of validity include *conclusion validity, internal validity, external validity*, and *construct validity*. Because many EBP teams do not have the skill set to judge the proper use of statistics in the studies under review, it is highly recommended that teams draw upon research texts, mentors, or experts to guide the process.

Conclusion Validity

Conclusion validity is the degree to which conclusions reached about relationships in the data are reasonable, believable, or credible. There are different reasons why conclusions about the existence of a relationship may be wrong. It is often hard to see a relationship because the measures used or observations made have low reliability (discussed later in the chapter), because the relationship being examined may be too weak, or because the sample size was too small to detect a relationship, even if one existed (Trochim, 2006).

When examining conclusion validity, the team should consider two types of error: Type I (finding statistical significance when no true difference exists) and Type II (failing to find statistical significance when a true difference exists). Type I error, also known as a false positive error, arises when the researcher concludes that differences between groups are significant when, in fact, they are not. Type II error, also known as false negative error, occurs when the null hypothesis (no significant differences between groups) is accepted as true, when, in fact, differences actually exist.

Internal Validity

Internal validity is the degree to which observed changes in the dependent variable are caused by the experimental treatment or intervention, rather than from other possible causes. An EBP team should question if evidence exists pointing to a competing explanation for observed results. Many threats to internal validity exist, all of which represent possible sources of bias. These include *investigator bias,* such as the Hawthorne Effect, in which subjects alter their behavior because they are participating in a study, not because of the research intervention;

attrition bias, in which loss of subjects during a study affects the representative nature of the sample; and *selection bias,* which affects all nonrandom samples.

External Validity

One of the main obstacles to translating EBP findings into practice is generalizability, or *external validity* (Metge, 2011). External validity refers to the likelihood that conclusions involving generalizations of research findings apply to other settings or samples. An EBP team should question the degree to which study conclusions may reasonably hold true for its particular patient population and setting. Do the investigators state the participation rates of subjects and settings? Do they explain the intended target audience for the intervention or treatment? How representative is the sample of the population of interest?

External validity is susceptible to three major threats; the researchers' generalization could be wrong in terms of person, place, or time—that is, they attempt to generalize findings from one group of persons to another, one clinical site to another, or one time to another in ways that may not be appropriate (Trochim, 2006).

Construct Validity

Construct validity concerns the measurement of variables, specifically the legitimacy of assuming that what the investigators are measuring actually measures the construct of interest. A construct is a way of defining something. Construct validity refers to how well you translate your ideas into measures (Trochim, 2006). EBP teams often encounter discussion of construct validity with respect to instruments used in research studies, in which case it refers to the degree to which the instrument measures the construct (or concept developed by the researcher) under investigation. If the investigators define a measure in a way that is very different from how other researchers define the same measure, then the construct validity is suspect (Garson, 2011). Questions a nurse may pose to get at threats to construct validity include, "Did the researcher do a good job of defining the constructs? When the researchers say that they are measuring what they call fatigue, is that what they are really measuring?"

Measures of Reliability

The concept of *reliability* is used to describe the consistency of a set of measurements or of an instrument used to measure a construct. The question that is asked is, "Can the results be replicated if the test is repeated?" Reliability, in essence, refers to the repeatability of a test. For example, variation in measurements may exist when nurses use patient care equipment such as blood pressure cuffs or glucometers. A number of factors can contribute to variation between measures and tests: intra-subject variation (variation within the individual test subjects); intra-observer variation (variation in the interpretation of test results by the same reader); and inter-observer variation (variation across those reading the test results; Gordis, 2009).

Measures of Precision

Precision language describes populations and characteristics of populations. An EBP team should be very familiar with measures of *central tendency* (mean, median, and mode) and *variation* (standard deviation). The *mean* denotes the average value and is used with interval level data. Although a good measure of central tendency in normal distributions, the mean is misleading in cases involving skewed (asymmetric) distributions and extreme scores. The *median,* the number that lies at the midpoint of a distribution of values, is less sensitive to extreme scores and, therefore, of greater use in skewed distributions. The *mode* is the most frequently occurring value and is the only measure of central tendency used with nominal (categorical) data. *Standard deviation* is a measure of variability that denotes the spread of the distribution, and indicates the average variation of values from the mean.

Another measure of precision is *statistical significance*. To say that a result is statistically significant is to say that it is unlikely to have occurred by chance. The classic measure of statistical significance, the *p-value*, is a probability range from 0 to 1. It assumes that the *null hypothesis* (no difference between two variables) is true, and, if the p-value is below the significance level, then the null hypothesis is rejected. The smaller the p-value (the closer it is to 0), the more likely the result is statistically significant and the more likely one can reject the null hypothesis. In nursing literature, statistical significance is generally set at $p < 0.05$. One limitation of restricting interpretation of research results to p-values is that the p-value is dichotomous, that is, it only tells the reader whether a finding is likely to have been due to chance or not. It does not give any information about the overall meaning of the findings to clinical practice.

The concept of statistical significance is an important one, but should not be confused with the concept of *clinical significance*. Just because results are statistically significant does not mean that they have practical application to patient care. Statistically significant results are more likely to have clinical significance, but this is not always the case. In the same way, results that are not statistically significant (because of small sample sizes, for example) can still have clinical importance. Statistical significance is influenced by sample size. If the sample is large enough, findings may reveal statistical significance that is really not clinically important. Many large clinical trials obtain a high level of statistical significance with very small differences between groups.

Although p-values are useful for investigators when planning how large a study needs to be to demonstrate a certain magnitude of effect, they fail to give clinicians the information about the range of values within which the true treatment effect is found (Montori et al., 2004). For this purpose, the confidence interval helps to specify precision.

What exactly is the *confidence interval* (CI)? This measure of precision is an estimate of a range of values within which the actual value lies. The CI contains an upper and lower limit. A 95% CI is the range of values within which an investigator can be 95% confident that the actual values in a given population fall between the lower and upper limits. Confidence intervals give an interval estimate in which, with hypothetical repetitions of the experiment, the population parameter can be expected to fall (Hayat, 2010). Consider a study on the effect of sucrose analgesia used to manage pain during venipucture in newborn screening (Taddio, Shah, & Katz, 2009). The researchers found that sucrose-treated infants had significantly lower pain scores during post-venipuncture diaper change than did water-treated infants (mean difference: -1.4 (95% CI: -2.4 to -0.4)). With repeated measurement of the population, the researchers would expect to find (with a 95% degree of certainty) consistent differences in neonatal pain scores, with the mean falling between -2.4 and -0.4.

The use of effect size contributes to the distinction between clinical and statistical significance. It is essential to the interpretation of results. An effect may be the result of a treatment, a decision, an intervention, or a program. Ellis (2010) postulates that the work of most researchers is to estimate the size of effects and cautions; that researchers must interpret not only the statistical significance of results, but also their practical application. The most commonly used effect size estimate is Cohen's *d*, whereby 0.8 is considered to be a large effect, 0.5 is interpreted as a medium effect, and 0.2 equates a small effect (Cohen, 1988). Mays & Melnyk (2009) recommend evaluating the effect size independently of the p-value. The effect size is a more precise measure of the treatment effect (difference in outcome between intervention groups) in the sample; whereas, the p-value can be affected by sample size. Consider that an experimental group of 20 new graduates are given a competency test on assessment of cardiac function after having a simulation experience. Their average score is 80, with a standard deviation of 10; the control group, which did not have a simulation experience, scores 75 with a standard deviation of 10. In this example of equal standard deviations and equal group sizes, the effect size is calculated as follows: 80 minus 75, divided by 10 (s) equals a 0.5 effect size; therefore, you have a medium effect size. The researcher may want to consider replicating the study with two other groups of new graduates to see if the same effect size is found.

Appraising the Strength and Quality of Research Evidence

The use of rating scales assists the critical appraisal of evidence. Rating scales present a structured way to differentiate evidence of varying strengths and quality. The underlying assumption is that recommendations from strong evidence of high quality would be more likely to represent best practices than evidence of lower strength and less quality. Tables 6.3 and 6.4 present the rating schemes used in the Johns Hopkins Nursing Evidence-based Practice (JHNEBP) process to evaluate the strength and quality of *research* evidence. (See also Appendix C).

Table 6.3   Strength of Research Evidence Rating Scheme

LEVEL	TYPE OF EVIDENCE
I	Evidence obtained from an experimental study, randomized controlled trial (RCT), or systematic review of RCTs, with or without meta-analysis
II	Evidence obtained from a quasi-experimental study or systematic review of a combination of RCTs and quasi-experimental studies, or quasi-experimental studies only, with or without meta-analysis
III	Evidence obtained from a quantitative non-experimental study; systematic review of a combination of RCTs, quasi-experimental, and non-experimental studies, or non-experimental studies only with or without meta-analysis; or qualitative study or systematic review of qualitative studies, with or without a meta-synthesis

Table 6.4   Quality Rating Scheme for Research Evidence

Grade	Research Evidence
A: High	Consistent, generalizable results; sufficient sample size for study design; adequate control; definitive conclusions; consistent recommendations based on comprehensive literature review that includes thorough reference to scientific evidence
B: Good	Reasonably consistent results; sufficient sample size for the study design; some control; fairly definitive conclusions; reasonably consistent recommendations based on fairly comprehensive literature review that includes some reference to scientific evidence
C: Low or Major flaw	Little evidence with inconsistent results; insufficient sample size for the study design; conclusions cannot be drawn

Grading Quality of Research Evidence

The large numbers of checklists and rating instruments available for grading the quality of research studies presents a challenge to an EBP team. Tools to appraise the quality of scientific evidence usually contain explicit criteria with varying degrees of specificity according to the evidence type. EBP teams often do not have the comprehensive knowledge of methodological strengths and limitations required to interpret these criteria. An EBP team needs to involve someone with knowledge of interpretation of research and statistics, often a nurse with a doctoral degree, to guide them through the process.

Because the development of any EBP skill set is evolutionary, the JHNEBP Model uses a broadly defined quality rating scale. This provides structure for the EBP team, yet allows for the application of critical-thinking skills specific to the team's knowledge and experience. The application of this scale, shown in Table 6.4, accommodates qualitative judgments related to both research and non-research evidence.

Judgments of quality should be relative. At any given point in the process, each individual or group applies the same interpretation to the body of evidence. As the group gains experience reading and appraising research, the members' comfort level in making this determination will likely improve.

Rating Strength of Research Evidence

Research evidence, when well-executed (of good to high quality), is generally given a higher strength rating than other types of evidence. When appraising individual research studies, three major components come into play: *study design*, which has been discussed as the level of evidence; *study quality*, which refers to study methods and execution, with particular attention to study limitations, and reflects the appraiser's confidence that the estimates of an effect are adequate to support recommendations (Balshem et al., 2011); and *directness*, or the extent to which subjects, interventions, and outcome measures are similar to those of interest.

When a team is appraising overall strength of evidence reviewed, a fourth component is added: *consistency,* or similarities in the size and/or direction of estimated effects across studies (Balshem et al., 2011). Identification of study designs and examination of *threats* to validity specific to the evidence type also help an EBP team to determine the overall strength and quality of research evidence.

Strength of Meta-analyses (Level I Evidence)

The strength of the evidence on which recommendations are made within a meta-analytic design depends on the type and quality of studies included in the meta-analysis as well the design of the meta-analysis itself. Factors to take into consideration include sampling criteria (primary studies included in the analysis), quality of the primary studies, and statistical heterogeneity (variability) of results across studies (Polit & Beck, 2008).

First, the EBP team needs to look at the types of research designs (level of evidence) included in the meta-analysis. The strongest meta-analyses contain only randomized controlled trials. Evidence from these studies is level I evidence. Some meta-analyses include data from quasi-experimental or non-experimental studies; hence, evidence would be a level commensurate with the lowest level of research design included (e.g., if the meta-analysis included experimental and quasi-experimental studies, then the meta-analysis would be level II).

Second, the team should look at the quality of studies included in the meta-analysis. For an EBP team to evaluate evidence obtained from a meta-analysis, the report of the meta-analysis must be detailed enough for the reader to understand the studies included.

Third, the team should assess the quality of the meta-analysis. Meta-analyses reports should clearly identify a focused research question; describe a systematic, reproducible literature search; identify a systematic process for study selection; detail characteristics and a quality assessment of all included studies; and report statistical methods used to combine studies (Hussain, Bookwala, Sancheti, & Bhandari, 2011).

Strength of Experimental Studies (Level I Evidence)

The strength of evidence is the highest, or level I, when derived from a well-designed RCT on the question of interest (see Table 6.3). Level I evidence is also derived from a meta-analysis of RCTs that support the same findings in different samples of the same population. Internal validity, discussed earlier in this chapter, refers to the extent to which inferences regarding cause and effect are true. Internal validity is relevant only to studies that try to establish causal relationships. Polit and Beck (2008, p. 295) write that "true experiments possess a high degree of internal validity because the use of manipulation and randomization usually enables the researcher to rule out most alternative explanations for the results." Potential threats to internal validity specific to experimental studies can be found in *bias*, or systematic error, in which the way the study was designed, conducted, or reported leads to conclusions that are systematically untrue and *random error*, which occurs due to chance variability in the measured data (Akobeng, 2008).

Types of bias include *selection bias, confounding, performance bias, detection bias,* and *attrition bias.*

- Although randomization is designed to eliminate *selection bias*, problems can occur during the randomization process itself (Akobeng, 2008). Questions an EBP team may pose to uncover potential selection bias include, "Did the authors clearly describe the method used to generate a random sequence of allocation by which to assign patients? Were people involved in subject recruitment blinded to the next treatment assignment? Did the researcher respect the assigned treatment or was the assignment altered?"

- *Confounding*, another type of bias that can occur in experimental studies, refers to situations in which a measure of the intervention's effect is distorted because of the association of the intervention with other factors that influence the outcome (Akobeng, 2008). For example, a decrease in length of stay on a unit that is studying the effects of multidisciplinary rounding may be affected by changes in insurance reimbursement rules. Though randomization attempts to balance known and unknown confounding factors, attempts to control for confounders are affected by sample size and baseline characteristics of the groups.

- When systematic variations exist in the care provided to subjects in the control group as compared with care provided to subjects in the intervention group, *performance bias* can occur. For example, in a study of wound care regimens, differences in mattress surfaces on the two units could have an effect on outcomes.

- When systematic variations exist between the two groups during outcome assessment, *detection bias* can occur (Akobeng, 2008). For example, if one study group is led by a certified wound care nurse and the other group is led by a senior staff nurse, then the group that has access to a higher level of expertise may be better able to evaluate outcomes than the group without such access. Another example of detection bias: researchers' perceptions of the efficacy of the intervention being tested or their knowledge of which treatment the patient is receiving (experiment or control) may have an influence on patient management during the trial. Under optimal circumstances, the researcher and the subjects are not aware of whether the subject has been randomized to the experimental group or the control group. This is *double-blinding*. For example, the subjects, their caregivers, or others involved in a study would not be told whether the subject is receiving a vitamin supplement or a placebo (inactive substance). This approach is an attempt to minimize bias on the part of subjects and researchers. Sometimes, it may be possible to blind the subjects to the experimental treatment, but not the investigator who applies either the experimental treatment or a control treatment (e.g., comparing two patient educational strategies). This is known as *single-blinding*.

- *Attrition bias* occurs when patients are withdrawn from the study because of deviations from protocol or are lost to follow-up (Akobeng, 2008). Patients who are excluded may not be representative of the subjects who continue in the study, so the analysis should include all of the patients randomized, whether or not they completed the study.

External validity refers to the extent that results will hold true across different subjects, settings, and procedures. The most frequent criticism by clinicians of RCTs is lack of external validity. Results from an RCT that has internal validity may be clinically limited if it lacks external validity, that is, if results cannot be applied to the relevant population. Potential threats to external validity in experimental studies relate to setting selection; patient selection; characteristics of randomized patients; the difference between the trial protocol and routine practices, outcome measures and follow-up; and adverse effects of the treatment (Rothwell, 2010). Questions a team may pose to uncover potential threats to external validity include, "How confident are we that the study findings can transfer from the sample to the entire population? Did subjects have inherent differences even before manipulation of the independent variable (selection bias)? Are participants responding in a certain way because they know they are being observed (the Hawthorne Effect)? Are there researcher behaviors or characteristics that may influence the subject's responses (experimenter effect)? In multi-institutional studies, are there variations in how study coordinators at various sites managed the trial? Has following subjects more frequently or having them take diagnostic tests affected the outcomes in unpredicted ways? Did the study have a high dropout rate, affecting the representative nature of the sample? Is the sample size adequate?"

Strength of Quasi-experimental Studies (Level II Evidence)

The strength of evidence gained from well-designed, quasi-experimental studies is lower than that of experimental studies. However, quasi-experimental studies are indicated when ethical considerations, practical issues, and feasibility prohibit the conduct of RCTs. For that reason, the strength of evidence rating for a well-designed quasi-experimental study is level II (See Table 6.3).

As with experimental studies, threats to internal validity for quasi-experimental studies include maturation, testing, and instrumentation, with the additional threats of history and selection (Polit & Beck, 2008). The occurrence of external events during the study (threat of history) can affect subject response to the investigational intervention or treatment. Additionally, when groups are not assigned randomly, the very nature of nonequivalent groups is such that pre-existing differences can affect the outcome. Questions the EBP team may pose to uncover potential threats to internal validity include, "Did some event occur during the course of the study that may have influenced the results of the study? Are there processes occurring within subjects over the course of the study because of the passage of time (maturation) rather than a result of the experimental intervention? Could the pre-test have influenced the subject's performance on the post-test? Were the measurement instruments and procedures the same for both points of data collection?"

In terms of external validity, threats associated with sampling design, such as patient selection and characteristics of nonrandomized patients, affect the general findings. External validity improves if the researcher uses random selection of subjects, even if random assignment to groups is not possible.

Strength of Non-Experimental and Qualitative Studies (Level III Evidence)

The strength of evidence gained from well-designed, non-experimental studies and qualitative studies is the lowest rung of the research evidence ladder (Level III), but is still higher than that of non-research evidence. Questions of internal validity do not apply when reviewing descriptive designs (quantitative or qualitative).

When looking for potential threats to external validity in quantitative non-experimental studies, the EBP team can pose the questions described under experimental and quasi-experimental studies. In addition, the team may ask further questions, such as, "Did the researcher attempt to control for extraneous variables with the use of careful subject selection criteria? Did the researcher attempt to minimize the potential for socially acceptable responses by the subject? Did the study rely on documentation as the source of data? In methodological studies (developing, testing, and evaluating research instruments and methods), were the test subjects selected from the population for which the test will be used? Was the survey response rate high enough to generalize findings to the target population? For historical research studies, are the data authentic and genuine?"

Qualitative studies offer many challenges with respect to the question of validity. A number of ways to determine validity in qualitative research have been postulated. Three common approaches are

- *Transactional validity*, an interactive process between researcher and subjects that uses such tools as trustworthiness, member checking, and triangulation
- *Transformational validity*, a progressive process that leads to social change and involves self-reflection and empathy on the part of the researcher while working with subjects

- *Holistic validity*, an open process that is narrative, nonjudgmental, uses more than one voice, and reflects on the validity of text and action (Cho & Trent, 2006).

Issues of validity in qualitative research are complex, so the EBP team should appraise how well the researcher(s) discuss how they determined validity for the particular study.

Strength of Meta-syntheses (Level III Evidence)

It is clear that evaluating and synthesizing qualitative research presents many challenges. It is not surprising that EBP teams may feel at a loss when it comes to assessing the quality of meta-synthesis. Approaching these reviews from a broad perspective enables the team to look for indicators of quality that both quantitative and qualitative summative research techniques have in common.

Explicit search strategies, inclusion and exclusion criteria, methodological details (not only of the included studies, but also of the conduct of the meta-synthesis itself), and reviewer management of study quality should all be noted. Similar to other summative modalities, a "meta-synthesis should be undertaken by a team of experts since the application of multiple perspectives to the processes of study appraisal, coding, charting, mapping, and interpretation may result in additional insights, and thus in a more complete interpretation of the subject of the review" (Jones, 2004, page 277).

EBP teams need to keep in mind that judgments related to study strengths and weaknesses, as well as to the suitability of recommendations for the target population are both context-specific and dependent on the question asked. Some conditions or circumstances, such as clinical setting or time of day, are relevant to determining the applicability of a particular recommended intervention.

Tips for Reading Research

Teams engaging in EBP activities should be educated readers and interpreters of research publications. The completeness of a research report and the reader's ability to understand the meaning of terms used in the report can help or hinder an EBP team's efforts. Though standards exist for writing research articles, the degree to which journals demand adherence to these standards varies. Classic elements of published research include the *title, abstract, introduction, method, results, discussion,* and *conclusion* (Lunsford & Lunsford, 1996). Readers will find that research reports do not always clearly delineate these sections with headers, although the elements may still be present. For example, typically the introduction or conclusion of a research report has no heading.

The Title

When searching for written research evidence, an EBP team encounters a listing of potential titles. The title presents a starting point in determining whether or not the article has potential to be included in an EBP review. Ideally, the title should be informative and help the reader understand what type of study is being reported. A well-chosen title states what was done, to whom it was done, and how it was done. Consider the title "Randomised Controlled Trial of a Family-led Mutual Support Programme for People with Dementia" (Wang & Chien, 2011). The reader is immediately apprised of what was done (family-led mutual support programme intervention), to whom it was done (people with dementia), and how it was done (a randomized controlled trial).

Often articles germane to an EBP question are skipped because the title does not give a clue as to its relevance. For example, consider the title "Urinary Tract Infection Rates Associated with Re-Use of Catheters in Clean Intermittent Catheterization of Male Veterans" (Kannankeril, Lam, Reyes, & McCartney, 2011). Although the reader can get the idea that the article concerns urinary tract infection rates in male veterans who undergo clean intermittent catheterization (*what* and *in whom*), the title does not give any indication that this is a report of a non-experimental research study using a descriptive design. The title is more reflective of an opinion piece than a research report.

The Abstract

The abstract is usually located after the title and author section and is graphically set apart by use of a box, shading, or italics. A good abstract contains information about a study's purpose, method, results, conclusions, and clinical relevance.

Huck (2004, p. 14) writes that "an abstract gives you a thumbnail sketch of a study, thus allowing you to decide whether the article fits into your area of interest," but cautions that a danger exists if a team thinks they can read only the abstract and forego reading the entire article. The abstract should serve as a screening device only.

The Introduction

If the abstract appears to be relevant, the team should move on then to an examination of the introduction. The introduction contains the background as well as a problem statement that tells why the investigators have chosen to conduct the particular study. Background is best presented within the context of a current literature review, and the author should identify the knowledge gap between what is known and what the study seeks to find out (or answer). A clear, direct statement of purpose should be included as well as a statement of expected results or hypotheses. The statement of purpose is often, although not always, located immediately before the article's first main heading.

The Conclusion

The conclusion should contain a brief restatement of the results and implications of the study (Lunsford & Lunsford, 1996). If the conclusion is not called out by a separate header, it usually falls at the end of the discussion section.

The Method

This section describes how a study is conducted (study procedures) in sufficient detail so that a reader can replicate the study, if desired. For example, if the intervention was administration of a placebo, the nature of the placebo should be stated. An investigator should identify the intended study population and provide a description of inclusion and exclusion criteria. How subjects were recruited and demographic characteristics of those who actually took part in the study should be included. In addition, if instrumentation was used, the method section should present evidence of instrument quality, even if well-known, published tools are used. Finally, the report should contain a description of how data were collected and analyzed.

The Results

Study results list the findings of the data analysis and should not contain commentary. Give particular attention to figures and tables, which are the heart of most papers. Look to see whether results report statistical versus clinical significance and look up unfamiliar terminology, symbols, or logic.

The Discussion

Results should be tied to material in the introduction. The research findings should be discussed and meaning given to the results. The main weaknesses or limitations of the study should be identified with the actions taken to minimize them, and the broad implications of the findings should be stated.

The reviewer should be cautioned that writers may use language to sway the reader. In his classic discussion on reading research, Graham (1957) notes that researchers can overstate their findings or use an assertive sentence in a way that makes their statement of findings sound like a well-established fact. (Critically view vague expressions similar to "It is generally believed that….").

The Overall Report

The parts of the research article should be highly interconnected and provide sufficient information so the reviewer can make an informed judgment about the connections. Any hypotheses should flow directly from the review of literature. Results should support arguments presented in the discussion and conclusion sections.

An EBP team should be aware of duplicate publications, that is, more than one publication that reports findings from the same research study. "Duplicate publication of original research is particularly problematic, since it can result in inadvertent double counting or inappropriate weighting of the results of a single study, which distorts the available evidence" (International Committee of Medical Journal Editors, 2010, IIID2).

A Practical Tool for Appraising Research Evidence

The Research Evidence Appraisal Tool (see Appendix E) gauges the strength and quality of research evidence. The front of the tool contains questions to guide the team in determining the level of strength of evidence and the quality of the primary studies included in the review. Strength is higher (level I) with evidence from at least one well-designed, randomized controlled trial (RCT) than from at least one well-designed quasi-experimental (level II), non-experimental (level III), or qualitative (level III) study. The reverse side of the tool contains questions specific to the study methods and execution to determine quality of the research.

An EBP team can use the Individual Evidence Summary Tool (see Appendix G) to summarize key findings from each of the individual pieces of evidence that answers the EBP question. This enables the team to view pertinent information related to each source (author, evidence type, sample type and size, setting, study findings that help answer the EBP question, limitations, level of evidence, and quality ratings) in one document.

An EBP team can use the Synthesis and Recommendations Tool (see Appendix H) to document the quantity or number of evidence sources for each level of evidence, determine the overall quality rating for each level, and synthesize findings to conclude if changes in processes or systems should be made. The team's final recommendations are listed at the bottom of the tool. A guide for how to synthesize evidence is provided in Appendix I, Synthesis of Evidence Guide.

Recommendation for Nurse Leaders

Knowledge gained from research studies is valuable only to the extent that it is shared with others and appropriately translated into practice. Professional standards have long held that nurses need to integrate the best available evidence, including research findings, into practice decisions. Research articles can be intimidating to novice and expert nurses alike. Reading scientific papers is "partly a matter of experience and skill, and partly learning the specific vocabulary of a field" (McNeal, 2005). Nurse leaders can best support EBP by providing clinicians with the knowledge and skills necessary to appraise research evidence.

Only through continuous learning can clinicians gain the confidence needed to incorporate evidence gleaned from research into the day-to-day care of individual patients.

Summary

This chapter arms EBP teams with practical information to guide the appraisal of research evidence, a task that often presents difficulties for non-researchers. An overview of the various types of research evidence is presented, including attention to individual research studies and summaries of multiple research studies. Tips for reading research reports are provided, along with guidance on how to appraise the strength and quality of research evidence.

References

Agency for Healthcare Research and Quality (AHRQ). (2011). Evidence-based practice centers. Retrieved from http://www.ahrq.gov/clinic/epc/

Akobeng, A. K. (2008). Assessing the validity of clinical trials. *Journal of Pediatric Gastroenterology and Nutrition, 47*(3), 277-282.

Allen, M. (2011). Violence and voice: Using a feminist constructivist grounded theory to explore women's resistance to abuse. *Qualitative Research, 11*(1), 23-45.

Balshem, H., Helfand, M., Schünemann, H. J., Oxman, A. D., Kunz, R., Brozek, J., … Guyatt, G. H. (2011). GRADE guidelines: 3. Rating the quality of evidence. *Journal of Clinical Epidemiology, 64*(4), 401-406.

Barnett-Page, E., & Thomas, J. (2009). Methods for synthesis of qualitative research: a critical review. *BMC Medical Research Methodology, 9,* (59).

Beauvais, A. M., Brady, N., O'Shea, E. R., & Griffin, M. T. (2011). Emotional intelligence and nursing performance among nursing students. *Nurse Education Today, 31*(4), 396-401.

Beck, C. T. (2009a). Metasynthesis: A goldmine for evidence-based practice. *AORN, 90*(5), 701-702, 705-710.

Beck, C. T. (2009b). Viewing the rich, diverse landscape of qualitative research. *Perioperative Nursing Clinics, 4*(3), 217-229.

Belli, G. (2009). Analysis and interpretation of nonexperimental studies. In S. D., Lapan, & M. T. Quartaroli, (Eds.). *Research Essentials: An Introductions to Designs and Practices* (pp. 59-77). Retrieved from http://media.wiley.com/product_data/excerpt/95/04701810/0470181095-1.pdf

Ceber, E., Turk, M., & Ciceklioglu, M. (2010). The effects of an educational program on knowledge of breast cancer, early detection practices, and health beliefs of nurses and midwives. *Journal of Clinical Nursing, 19*(15-16), 2363-2371.

Chazelle, E., Lemogne, C., Morgan, K., Kelleher, C. C., Chastang, J. F., & Niedhammer, I. (2011). Explanations of educational differences in major depression and generalised anxiety disorder in the Irish population. *Journal of Affective Disorders*, *134*(1-3), 304-314. June 14, Epub ahead of print.

Cho, J., & Trent, A. (2006). Validity in qualitative research revisited. *Qualitative Research*, *6*(3), 319-340.

Chong, P. H., Poon, W. H. (2011). The lived experience of palliative homecare nurses in Singapore. *Singapore Medical Journal, 52*(3), 151-157.

The Cochrane Collaboration. (2010a). The Cochrane Collaboration. Working together to provide the best evidence in health care. Retrieved from http://www.cochrane.org/

The Cochrane Collaboration. (2010b). Cumulative meta-analysis. Retrieved from http://www.cochrane.org/glossary/5

Cohen, J. (1988). *Statistical power analysis for the behavioral sciences.* New York: Academic Press.

Dybitz, S. B., Thompson, S., Molotsky, S., & Stuart, B. (2011). Prevalence of diabetes and the burden of comorbid conditions among elderly nursing home patients. *American Journal of Geriatric Pharmacotherapy*, *9*(4), 212-223.

Ellis, P. D. (2010). Effect sizes and the interpretation of research results in international business. *Journal of International Studies*, *41*, 1581-1588.

Fouquier, K. F. (2011). The concept of motherhood among three generations of African-American women. *Journal of Nursing Scholarship*, *43*(2), 145-153.

Garson, G. D. (2011). *PA 765. Statnotes. Topics in multivariate analysis.* Retrieved from http://faculty.chass.ncsu.edu/garson/PA765/statnote.htm

Gliner, J. A., Morgan, G. A., & Leech, N. L. (2009). *Research methods in applied settings: An integrated approach to design and analysis* (2nd ed.). London: Taylor & Francis Group.

Gordis, L. (2009). *Epidemiology.* Philadelphia, PA: Saunders Elsevier.

Graham, C. D., (1957). A dictionary of useful research phrases. Originally published in *Metal Progress.* 71(5). Retrieved from http://www.ece.vt.edu/thou/Dictionary%20of%20Useful%20Research%20Phrases.htm

Hayat, M. (2010). Understanding statistical significance. *Nursing Research,* *59*(3), 219-223.

Higgins. J. P. T., & Green, S. (Eds.). *Cochrane handbook for systematic reviews of interventions,* (Version 5.1.0 [Updated March 2011]). The Cochrane Collaboration, 2011. Retrieved from www.cochrane-handbook.org

Hill, K. S. (2011). Work satisfaction, intent to stay, desires of nurses and financial knowledge among bedside and advance practice nurses. *Journal of Nursing Administration*, *41*(5), 211-217.

Huck, S. W. (2004). *Reading statistics and research* (4th ed.). Boston, MA: Pearson Allyn and Bacon.

Hussain, N., Bookwala, A., Sancheti, P., & Bhandari, M. (2011). The 3-minute appraisal of a meta-analysis. *Indian Journal of Orthopaedics, 45*(1), 4-5.

International Committee of Medical Journal Editors. (2010). *Uniform requirements for manuscripts submitted to biomedical journals: Writing and editing for biomedical publications.* Retrieved from http://www.ICMJE.org

Jones, K. R. (2010). Rating the level, quality, and strength of the research evidence. *Journal of Nursing Care Quality. 25*(4), 304-312.

Jones, M. L. (2004). Application of systematic review methods to qualitative research: Practical issues. *Journal of Advanced Nursing, 48*(3), 271-278.

Jones, D., Duffy, M. E., & Flanagan, J. (2011). Randomized clinical trial testing efficacy of a nurse-coached intervention in arthroscopy patients. *Nursing Research, 60*(2), 92-99.

Kannankeril, A. J., Lam, H. T., Reyes, E. B., & McCartney, J. (2011). Urinary tract infection rates associated with re-use of catheters in clean intermittent catheterization of male veterans. *Urologic Nursing, 31*(1), 41-48.

Knowles, A. (2011). Resilience among Japanese atomic bomb survivors. *International Nursing Review, 58*(1), 54-60.

Lu, C. Y. (2009). Observational studies: A review of study designs, challenges, and strategies to reduce confounding. *The International Journal of Clinical Practice, 63*(5), 691-697.

Lunsford, T. R., & Lunsford, B. R. (1996). Research forum: How to critically read a journal research article. *Journal of Prosthetics and Orthotics, 8*(1), 24-31.

Mays, M. Z., & Melnyk, B. M. (2009). A call for reporting of effect sizes in research reports to enhance critical appraisal and evidence-based practice. *Worldviews on Evidence-Based Nursing, 6*(3), 125-129.

Mazanec, S. R., Daly, B. J., Douglas, S., & Musil, C. (2011). Predictors of psychosocial adjustment during the post-radiation treatment transition. *Western Journal of Nursing Research, 33*(4), 540-559.

McHugh, M. D., Shang, J., Sloane, D. M., & Aiken, L. H. (2011). Risk factors for hospital-acquired "poor glycemic control": A case-control study. *International Journal for Quality in Health Care, 23*(1), 44-51.

McNeal, A. (2005). How to read a scientific research paper—A four-step guide for students and for faculty. Retrieved from http://helios.hampshire.edu/~apmNS/design/RESOURCES/HOW_READ.html

Metge, C. J. (2011). What comes after producing the evidence? The importance of external validity in translating science to practice. *Clinical Therapeutics, 33*(5), 578-580.

Moher, D., Liberati, A., Tetzlaff, J., Altman, D. G., & PRISMA Group. (2009). Preferred reporting items for systematic reviews and meta-analyses the PRISMA statement. *Journal of Clinical Epidimiology, 62*(10), 1006-1012.

Montori, V. M., Kleinbart, J., Newman, T. B., Keitz, S., Wyer, P. C., Moyer, V., & Guyatt, G., for the Evidence-Based Medicine Teaching Tips Working Group. (2004). Tips for learners of evidence-based medicine: 2. Measures of precision (confidence intervals). *Canadian Medical Association Journal, 171*(6), 611-615.

Noblit, G. W., & Hare, R. D. (1988). *Meta-ethnography: Synthesizing qualitative studies.* Newbury Park, CA: Sage.

Palumbo, M. V., Marth, N., & Rambur, B. (2011). Advanced practice registered nurse supply in a small state: Trends to inform policy. *Policy, Politics, & Nursing Practice, 12*(1):27-35 May 25, ePub ahead of print.

Polit, D. F., & Beck, C. T. (2008). *Nursing research: Generating and assessing evidence for nursing practice* (8th ed.). Philadelphia: Lippincott Williams & Wilkens.

Roberts, C. A. (2010). Unaccompanied hospitalized children: A review of the literature and incidence study. *Journal of Pediatric Nursing, 25*(6), 470-476.

Rothwell, P. M. (2010). Commentary: External validity of results of randomized trials: Disentangling a complex concept. *International Journal of Epidemiology, 39*(1), 94-96.

Ruffin, P. T. (2011). A history of massage in nurse training school curricula (1860-1945). *Journal of Holistic Medicine, 29*(1), 61-67.

Schmied, V., Beake, S., Sheehan, A., McCourt, C., & Dykes, F. (2011). Women's perceptions and experiences of breastfeeding support: A metasynthesis. *Birth, 38*(1), 49-60.

Schmid, A., Hoffman, L., Happ, M. B., Wolf, G. A., & DeVita, M. (2007). Failure to rescue: A literature review. *Journal of Nursing Administration, 37*(4), 188-198.

Sigma Theta Tau International. (2011). *Worldviews on evidence-based nursing.* Retrieved from http://onlinelibrary.wiley.com/journal/10.1111/(ISSN)1741-6787

Sword, W., Landy, C. K., Thabane, L., Watt, S., Krueger, P., Farine, D., & Foster, G. (2011). Is mode of delivery associated with postpartum depression at 6 weeks: A prospective cohort study. *BJOG: An International Journal of Obstetrics and Gynaecology, 118*(8), 966-977.

Taddio, A., Shah, V., & Katz, J. (2009). Reduced infant response to a routine care procedure after sucrose analgesia. *Pediatrics, 123*(3), e425-e429.

Tavares de Souza, M., Dias da Silva, M., & de Carvalho, R. (2010). Integrative review: What is it? How to do it? *Einstein, 8*(1 Pt 1), 102-106.

Trochim, W. M. K. (2006). The Research Methods Knowledge Base. (2nd ed). Retrieved from http://www.socialresearchmethods.net/kb/ (version current as of August 10, 2006).

van Manen, M. (1997). Researching lived experience: Human science for an action sensitive pedagogy (2nd ed.). London, Canada: The Althouse Press.

Wang, L. Q., & Chien, W. T. (2011). Randomised controlled trial of a family-led mutual support programme for people with dementia. *Journal of Clinical Nursing, 20*(15-16), 2362-2366.

Werner, R. A., Gell, N., Hartigan, A., Wiggermann, N., & Keyserling, M. (2011). Risk factors for hip problems among assembly plant workers. *Journal of Occupational Rehabilitation, 21*(1), 84-89.

Wu, L., Forbes, A., Griffiths, P., Milligan, P., & While, A. (2010). Telephone follow-up to improve glycaemic control in patients with Type 2 diabetes: Systematic review and meta-analysis of controlled trials. *Diabetic Medicine*, 27(11), 1217-1225.

Yoo, H., Kim, S., Hur, H. K., & Kim, H. S. (2011). The effects of an animation distraction intervention on pain response of preschool children during venipuncture. *Applied Nursing Research*, 24(2), 94-100.

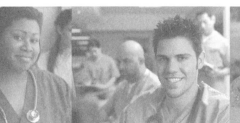
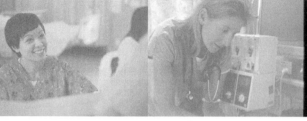

Evidence Appraisal: Non-Research

Sarah J. M. (Jodi) Shaefer, PhD, RN

Hayley D. Mark, PhD, MPH, RN

One of the distinguishing features of EBP is the inclusion of the multiple sources of evidence. When research evidence does not exist or is insufficient to answer the practice question, nurses have a range of non-research evidence to draw from that has the potential to inform their practice.

Such evidence includes personal, aesthetic, and ethical ways of knowing (Carper, 1978), for example, the expertise, experience, and values of individual practitioners, patients and their families. For the purposes of this chapter, non-research study evidence is divided into summaries of evidence (clinical practice guidelines, consensus or position statements, literature reviews); organizational experience (quality improvement and financial and program evaluation data); expert opinion (individual(s) commentary or opinion, case reports); community standards; clinician experience; and consumer preferences. This chapter

- Describes types of non-research evidence
- Describes strategies for evaluating such evidence

- Recommends approaches for building nurses' capacity to appraise non-research evidence to inform their practice

Summaries of Research Evidence

Summaries of research evidence such as clinical practice guidelines, consensus or position statements, or literature reviews are excellent sources of evidence relevant to practice questions. These forms of evidence review and synthesize all research (not just experimental studies). However, they are not classified as research evidence because summaries of research evidence are often not comprehensive, and may not include an appraisal of study quality.

Clinical Practice Guidelines and Consensus/Position Statements

Clinical practice guidelines (CPGs) are systematically developed statements that guide clinical practice and evidence-based decision-making (Polit & Beck, 2010). They are recommendations that synthesize available experimental and clinical evidence with bedside experience and are open to comment, criticism, and updating (Deresinski & File, 2011). Consensus or position statements (CSs) are similar to CPGs in that they are systematically developed recommendations that may or may not be supported by research. CSs are broad statements of best practice, are most often meant to guide members of a professional organization in decision-making, and do not provide specific algorithms for practice (Lopez-Olivio, Kallen, Ortiz, Skidmore, & Suarez-Almazor, 2008).

The last two decades have seen an exponential increase in CPGs and CSs. To help practitioners determine the quality of CPGs, the Institute of Medicine identified eight desirable attributes, which include validity, reliability and reproducibility, clinical applicability, clinical flexibility, clarity, documentation, development by a multidisciplinary process, and plans for review (IOM, 1992). Many of these attributes were absent from published guidelines, resulting in the *Conference on Guideline Standardization* to promote guideline quality and to facilitate implementation (Shiffman et al., 2003). The *Appraisal of Guidelines Research and Evaluation (AGREE) Collaboration*, using a guideline appraisal instrument with documented reliability and validity, found that the availability of background information was the strongest predictor of guideline quality and that high-quality guidelines were more often produced by government-supported organizations or a structured, coordinated program (Fervers et al., 2005).

The National Guideline Clearinghouse (NGC), an initiative of the Agency for Healthcare Research and Quality (AHRQ), U.S. Department of Health and Human Services, has developed criteria designed to ensure rigor in developing and maintaining published guidelines (NGC, 2011). Included in these criteria are requirements that the clinical practice guideline

- Include systematically developed statements that contain recommendations, strategies, or information that assists health care practitioners and patients in making decisions
- Be officially sponsored by one or more medical specialty associations, relevant professional societies, public or private organizations, government agencies, or health care organizations or plans
- Have a corroborative, verifiable documentation of a systematic literature search and review of existing research evidence published in peer reviewed journals
- Have been developed, reviewed, or revised in the last 5 years and be available in print or electronic form in the English language

These rigorous standards are one of the reasons why the NGC is an excellent source of high quality guidelines. An example of a set of guidelines that meets the exacting requirements of the NGC is "Effectiveness-based Guidelines for the Prevention of Cardiovascular Disease in Women—2011 Update" (Mosca et al., 2011).

Despite these recommendations, guidelines still vary greatly in how they are developed and how the results are reported (Kuehn, 2011). In response to concern about the quality, two reports were released by the IOM to set standards for clinical practice guidelines (IOM, 2011). The IOM developed eight standard practices for creating CPGs (see Table 7.1). These standards describe the information that should be in the guidelines and the development processes that should be followed.

Table 7.1   Clinical Practice Guideline (CPG) Standards and Description

Standard	Description
Establish transparency	Funding and development process should be publicly available.
Disclose conflict(s) of interest (COI)	Individuals who create guidelines and panel chairs should be free from conflicts of interest. Funders are excluded from CPG development. All COI of each Guideline Development Group member should be disclosed.
Balance membership of guideline development group	Guideline developers should include multiple disciplines, patients, patient advocates, or patient consumer organizations.
Use systematic reviews	CPG developers should use systematic reviews that meet Institute of Medicine (IOM) standards.
Establish evidence foundations and rate strength of recommendations	Rating has specified criteria for strength of recommendations.
Articulate recommendations	Recommendations should follow a standard format and be worded so that compliance can be evaluated.
Include external reviewers	External reviews should represent all relevant stakeholders, and their identity should be keep confidential. A draft of the CPG should be available to the public at the external review stage or directly afterward.
Update guidelines	CPG should be updated when new evidence suggests the need, and CPG publication date, date of systematic evidence review, and proposed date for future review should be documented.

Literature Reviews

Literature review is a broad term that generally refers to a summary of published literature without systematic appraisal of evidence quality or strength. Traditional literature reviews are not confined to summaries of scientific literature; they can also present a narrative description of information from nonscientific literature, including reports of organizational experience and opinions of experts. Such reviews possess some of the desired attributes of a systematic review, but not the same standardized approach, appraisal, and critical review of the studies. For example, an author of a narrative review of research studies related to a particular question may describe comprehensive, even replicable, literature search strategies but neglect to appraise the quality of the studies discussed. Literature reviews also vary in completeness and often lack the intent of summarizing all the available evidence on a topic (Grant & Booth, 2009).

An example of a narrative literature review is "The Role of Simulation for Learning within Pre-registration Nursing Education—A Literature Review" (Ricketts, 2011), which draws information from published studies and reports of competencies, knowledge, and skills required by forensic mental health nurses.

Interpreting Evidence from Summaries of Research Evidence

Despite efforts to ensure quality, the degree to which CPGs and CSs draw from existing evidence can fluctuate. Most guidelines are based on systematic reviews developed by experts whose charge is to arrive at specific clinical conclusions (IOM, 2001). Additionally, guidelines can lack the specificity needed to ensure consistent application across patients with the same clinical situation. Because the evidence base can be limited or conflicting, the EBP team needs to exercise critical thinking and judgment when making recommendations.

In response to concerns about the methodological quality of CPGs, an international collaboration developed the AGREE Instrument (http:///www.agreetrust. org/about-agree/introduction0/), a 23-item assessment tool and users manual (The AGREE Research Trust, 2009; Brouwers et al., 2010). Key identifiers of CPG quality are scope and purpose, stakeholder involvement, rigor of development, clarity and presentation, applicability, and editorial independence (Singleton & Levin, 2008).

Recently, attention has been paid to assessing equity in clinical practice guidelines. Equity concerns arise in groups potentially vulnerable to inequity because of residence, race, occupation, gender, religion, education, socioeconomic status, social network, and capital (Dans et al., 2007). When appropriate, an EBP team must consider the sociopolitical dimensions of applying CPGs to disadvantaged patient populations.

The age of the patient population is equally as important. Consider the anatomic, physiologic, and developmental differences between children and adults before applying published guidelines. For example, Baharestani and Ratliff (2007) noted that many pressure ulcer prevention protocols for neonates and children have been extrapolated from adult practice guidelines, raising concerns about whether the needs of pediatric patients at risk for pressure ulcers have been adequately addressed.

EBP teams also need to note that although groups of experts create these guidelines which frequently carry a professional society's seal of approval, opinions that convert data to recommendations require subjective judgments that, in turn, leave room for error and bias (Detsky, 2006). Potential conflicts of interest can be generated by financial interests, job descriptions, personal research interests, and previous experience. The recent IOM panel recommended that whenever possible, individuals who create the guidelines should be free from conflicts of interest; if that is not possible, however, those individuals with conflicts of interest should make up a minority of the panel and should not serve as chair or cochair (IOM, 2011).

Key elements to note when examining the strength and quality of Level IV evidence are identified in Table 7.2 and in the JHNEBP Non-Research Evidence Appraisal Tool (see Appendix F). Given the lack of comprehensiveness of many literature reviews, the attributes listed in Table 7.1 apply differently to clinical practice guidelines and consensus statements than to literature reviews.

Table 7.2   Desirable Attributes of Summative Documents Used to Answer an EBP Question

Attribute	Description
Applicability to phenomenon of interest	Does the summative document address the particular practice question of interest (same population, same setting)?
Comprehensiveness of search strategy	Do the authors identify search strategies that move beyond the typical databases, such as MEDLINE and CINAHL?
	Are published and unpublished works included?
Clarity of method	Do the authors clearly specify how decisions were made to include and exclude studies from the analysis and how data were analyzed?
Unity and consistency of findings	Is there cohesive organization of study findings so that meaningful separation and synthesis of relevant concepts is clear to the reader?
	Does the publication contain logically organized tables with consistent information relative to the applicability of findings?
Management of study quality	Do the authors clearly describe how the review manages study quality?
Transparency of limitations	Are methodological limitations disclosed?
Believability of conclusions	Do the conclusions appear to be based on the evidence and capture the complexity of the clinical phenomenon?
Collective expertise	Was the review and synthesis done by a single individual with expertise or a group of experts?

Adapted from Whittemore (2005), Conn (2004), and Stetler et al., (1998).

Organizational Experience

Organizational experience often takes the form of quality improvement (QI) and financial or program evaluations. These sources of evidence can occur at any level in the organization and can be internal to an EBP team's organization or published reports from external organizations. Although they may be conducted within a framework of scientific inquiry and designed as research studies, most internal program evaluations are less rigorous (Level V). Frequently, they comprise pre- and/or post-implementation data at the organizational level accompanied by qualitative reports of personal satisfaction with the program. An example of a program evaluation is "Improving Teaching Strategies in an Undergraduate Community Health Nursing (CHN) Program: Implementation of a Service-Learning Preceptor Program" (Kazemi, Behan, & Boniauto, 2011), which evaluated a new program of service learning for community health students. This post-test-only method included time saved by preceptors, improved satisfaction of nursing students, and experiential learning for students.

Quality Improvement Reports

Quality improvement (QI) is a term that can be used interchangeably with quality management, performance improvement, total quality management, and continuous quality improvement (Yoder-Wise, 2011). These terms refer to ongoing efforts to improve the quality of care delivery and outcomes within an organization. QI is a cyclical method to examine workflows, processes, or systems within a specific organization. This information usually cannot be generalized beyond the organization. The organizational experience described here is distinctly different from quality-focused research or health services research intended to generalize results. Health services research uses experimental, quasi-experimental, or non-experimental research designs (described in Chapter 6) and should be reviewed and appraised accordingly.

QI is a method of self-examination to inform improvement efforts at the local level. During their review of non-research evidence, an EBP team should examine internal QI data relating to the practice question as well as QI initiatives based on similar questions published by peer institutions. As organizations become more mature in their QI efforts, they become more rigorous in the approach, the analysis of results, and the use of established measures as metrics (Newhouse, Pettit, Poe, & Rocco, 2006). In contrast to research studies, the findings from quality improvement studies are not meant to be generalized to other settings. Organizations that may benefit from the findings need to make decisions regarding implementation based on the characteristics of their organization.

QI reporting is an internal process; nevertheless, the desire to share the results from such projects is evident in the growing number of collaborative efforts targeting particular risk-prone issues. For example, the Institute of Healthcare Improvement (IHI) sponsors a learning and innovation network of quality-focused organizations working together to achieve improvement in health care areas such as perinatal care and the reduction of rehospitalization. The IHI expanded these efforts and is working across organizational boundaries and engaging payers, state and national policymakers, patients and families, and caregivers at multiple care sites and clinical interfaces through the *STate Action on Avoidable Rehospitalizations (STAAR) Initiative* (IHI, 2011). Results of these activities are presented at conferences and seminars, providing others the opportunity to learn about the latest improvement ideas. Although evidence obtained from QI initiatives is not as strong as that obtained through scientific inquiry, the sharing of successful QI stories has the potential to identify future EBP questions, QI projects, or research studies external to the organization.

An example of a quality improvement project is reported from an emergency department (ED) in Utah (Henderson, 2010). Emergency department staff tracked the unit's compliance with the IHI "Sepsis Resuscitation Bundle." The ED reduced the severe sepsis and shock mortality by 50% by improving specific processes that were unique to their ED. This Level V evidence is from one institution that implemented a quality improvement project.

Financial Evaluation

Financial and quality measures in health care facilities provide data to assess the cost associated with practice changes. Cost savings can be powerful information as the best practice is examined. An EBP team can find reports of cost-effectiveness and economic evaluations (Level V) in published data or internal organizational reports. The "Support Surfaces and Pressure Ulcers" EBP project you can read about in Chapter 10 is an example of a cost analysis with the rationale for changing all mattresses. This internal report was generated to determine potential cost savings and was used exclusively at one organization.

Terms used in the literature for projects dealing with finances include an *economic evaluation* that applies analytic techniques to identify, measure, and compare the costs and outcomes of two or more alternative programs or interventions (CDC, 2007). A common economic evaluation of health care decision-making is a *cost effectiveness analysis*, which compares costs of alternative interventions that produce a common health outcome. Although results of such an analysis can provide justification for a program, empirical evidence can provide support for an increase in program funding or a switch from one program to another (CDC, 2007). Polit and Beck (2010) provide other economic terms:

- **Cost analysis:** Analysis between cost and outcome for alternative interventions

- **Cost benefit:** Converts all costs and benefits of a program into dollars, allowing comparison of programs in monetary terms

- **Cost utility:** A special variant of cost effectiveness analysis that allows for the comparison of programs that address different health problems (e.g., breast cancer screening and diabetes control) because the outcomes are converted into a common health metric, such as quality-adjusted life years

Financial data can be evaluated as listed on the JHNEBP Non-Research Evidence Appraisal Tool (see Appendix F). In reviewing a report, examine the aim, method, measures, results, and discussion for clarity. Carande-Kulis et al. (2003) recommend that standard inclusion criteria for economic studies have an analytic method and provide sufficient detail regarding the method and results. In assessing the quality of the economic study, the Community Guide "Economic Evaluation Abstraction Form" (2010) suggests that you ask the following questions:

- Was the study population well-described?

- Was the question being analyzed well-defined?

- Did the study define the time frame?

- Were data sources for all costs reported?

- Were data sources and costs appropriate with respect to the program and population being tested?

- Was the primary outcome measure clearly specified?

- Did outcomes include the effects or unintended outcomes of the program?

- Was the analytic model reported in an explicit manner?

- Were sensitivity analyses performed?

Not all studies that include cost analysis are strictly financial evaluations. When evaluating an article with a cost analysis, note that some may be research and should be appraised using the Research Evidence Appraisal Tool (see Appendix E). For example, Sise et al. (2011) report findings on staffing costs, nurse-patient ratios, patient acuity, and outcomes over a 4-year period. Results indicated that patient volume increased and outcomes improved while patient acuity remained stable. After a review of this study, the EBP team would discover that this was actually a descriptive, longitudinal, non-experimental design study using comparative data analysis among years. Thus, it requires use of research appraisal criteria to judge the strength and quality of evidence.

Expert Opinion

The opinions of experts take the form of commentary articles, position statements, case reports, or letters to the editor. External recognition (state, regional, national, international) that a professional is an expert is critical to determining the confidence an EBP team has in the expert's recommendations. Assessing expertise of an author of commentaries and opinion pieces requires another step. The EBP team can review the author's education, work, university affiliations, publications on the topic; if others have cited the author's work; or if the author is a recognized speaker. For example, Lach (2010) provides an expert opinion on patient falls and challenges for nursing administrators. This article could be rated high quality because the author is on the faculty of a school of nursing and has additional publications on this topic. Her report is based on the literature with data supporting her opinion.

Case Report

A case report is an in-depth look at a single person, group, or other social unit to obtain a wealth of descriptive information to understand issues important to the phenomenon under study (Polit & Beck, 2010). It can be quantitative or qualitative in nature, and describes an individual case or a *case study*. "Direct Care Workers' Response to Dying and Death in the Nursing Home: A Case Study" (Black & Rubinstein, 2005) describes a sub-study of a multiyear, multi-site ethnographic study that used interviews, informal conversations, and on-site observations. This is a rigorous report of workers' experiences. The literature also includes cases of a single patient. "Returning to Work with Aphasia: A Case Study" (Morris, Franklin, & Menger, 2011) contains details on a single patient. These reports present a summary of anecdotal descriptions of a particular patient care scenario. Case reports provide insight into an individual case that may provide an alternative explanation or challenge current generalizations based on other types of research (Polit & Beck, 2010). Though the case report can provide the EBP team with insights into a specific clinical situation, it has limited generalizability and therefore is level V evidence.

Community Standard

When an EBP team is searching for evidence, one consideration is the current practice standard in the community. To learn the community standard, the EBP team identifies health care providers, agencies, or organizations for evidence. The team devises a standard list of questions and a systematic approach to data collection. For example, Johns Hopkins University School of Nursing students were assisting with an EBP project with the question "Does charge nurse availability during the shift affect staff nurse satisfaction with work flow?" An EBP team member contacted local hospitals to determine if charge nurses had patient assignments. Students developed a data sheet with questions about the health care facility, the unit, staffing pattern, and staff comments about satisfaction. The students reported the number of units contacted and responses, information source, and number of sources using the Non-Research Evidence Appraisal Tool. Additionally, this approach provides an opportunity to network with other clinicians about a clinical issue.

Social networking, blogs from a professional organization's websites, and special interest groups are another source of information about community standards. The Pediatric Emergency Medicine Database (http://www.pemdatabase.org/) is an online database that provides articles and a discussion list for clinical questions. These types of databases can provide helpful information about community standards.

Clinician Experience

Though this section focuses on nurse experience, the best application of EBP occurs within the interdisciplinary care team because no one discipline provides health care in isolation.

The concept of holistic care as the hallmark of nursing expertise, advocated by Benner (2001), supports the notion that evidence of all types (both research and non-research) must inform nursing practice. Novice nurses rely heavily on guidelines and care protocols to enhance skill development, looking at the patient as the sum of composite parts. The more experienced expert nurse has gained a grasp of each clinical situation and looks at each aspect of care as it pertains to the whole patient (Christensen & Hewitt-Taylor, 2006).

Clinical expertise (level V), both skill proficiency and professional judgment, is gained through the combination of education and clinical experiences. Personal judgments arising from past and present nurse-patient interactions, and knowledge about what works within the organization or system, adds depth to that expertise. Nurses who practice within an evidence-based framework are committed to personal growth, reflection, self-evaluation, accountability, and lifelong learning (Dale, 2006).

The Expertise in Practice Project (Hardy, Titchen, Manley, & McCormack, 2006) in the United Kingdom identified and examined attributes of nurse expertise and enabling factors. Attributes of expertise included

- **Holistic practice knowledge:** Drawing from a range of knowledge bases to inform action

- **Skilled know-how:** Enabling others by sharing knowledge and skills

- **Saliency:** Observing non-verbal cues to understand each individual's unique situation

- **Moral agency:** Consciously promoting each individual's dignity, respect, and individuality

- **Knowing the patient/client:** Promoting patient decision-making within the context of each individual's unique perspective

Enabling factors for nursing expertise included

- **Reflectivity:** The ability to continually reconsider, reassess, and reframe one's work

- **Organization of practice:** Organization and prioritization of workload

- **Autonomy and authority:** Taking responsibility for consequence of difficult decisions

- **Good interpersonal relationships:** Intentional in relationships

- **Recognition from others:** Regular feedback and acknowledgement of work

EBP team members can survey their internal and external organizational peers to obtain clinician expertise. For example, in the "Support Surfaces and Pressure Ulcers" exemplar (Chapter 10), the team describes their survey of wound care nurses and the data obtained on the current usage and recommended sleep surfaces for high-risk patients.

Patient/Consumer Preferences

Patients are consumers of health care and the term *consumer* also refers to a larger group of individuals using health services in a variety of settings. The art of nursing recognizes that humans are active participants in their life and make choices regarding their health (Milton, 2007). Health is a quality of life and is best described by the person who is experiencing it. Patient experience (level V) is a core component of a patient-centered approach to care, honoring lived experiences as evidence so the patient can be an active partner in decision-making. This is based on the core ethical value of respect for persons. Each patient has personal, religious, and cultural beliefs to account for that enable the individual to make informed care decisions. Individuals and families of different cultures, races, social, and economic classes are likely to have very dissimilar experiences with the health care system and, hence, have dissimilar perspectives on evidence-based practices (Birkel, Hall, Lane, Cohan, & Miller, 2003).

The expert nurse incorporates patient preferences into clinical decision-making by asking the following questions:

- Are the research findings and non-research evidence relevant to this particular patient's care?
- Have all care and treatment options based on the best available evidence been presented to the patient?
- Has the patient been given as much time as is necessary to allow for clarification and consideration of options?
- Have the patient's expressed preferences and concerns been considered when planning care?

The answer to these questions requires ethical practice and respect for a patient's autonomy. Combining sensitivity to individual patient needs and thoughtful application of best evidence leads to optimal patient-centered outcomes.

Patients/consumers play a key role in managing their care. As consumer-driven health care has expanded, recent reports recommend specific efforts for consumer education and improving health literacy (Weaver, 2010). Nurses are increasingly cognizant of the critical role the consumer plays in the quality and safety of health care. Upholding the belief that consumer preferences and values are integral to EBP, Melnyk and Fineout-Overholt (2006) offered three suggestions to involve patients in clinical decision-making: (a) respect patient participation in clinical decision-making, (b) assess patient preferences and values during the admission intake process, and (c) provide patient education about treatment plan options. Additionally, providing information to patients about best practice recommendations as these apply to their particular clinical situation is important. Only an informed patient can truly participate in clinical decision-making, ensuring the best possible outcomes of care.

Engaging consumers of health care in EBP goes well beyond the individual patient encounter. Consumer organizations can play a significant role in supporting implementation and promulgation of EBP. Consumer-led activities can take the form of facilitating research to expedite equitable adoption of new and existing best practices, promoting policies for the development and use of advocacy tool kits, and influencing provider adoption of EBP (Birkel, Hall, Lane, Cohan, & Miller 2003). In examining the information provided by consumers, the EBP team should consider the credibility of the individual or group. What segment and volume of the consumer group do they represent? Do their comments and opinion provide any insight into the team's EBP question?

An EBP team should take into consideration the perspectives of children, young families, the elderly, and aging families. They should ascertain whether suggested recommendations have been designed and developed with sensitivity and knowledge of diverse cultural groups.

Recommendations for Nurse Leaders

Time and resource constraints compel nurse leaders to find creative ways to support integration of new knowledge into clinical practice. The time the average staff nurse has to devote to gathering and appraising evidence is limited. Therefore, finding the most efficient way to gain new knowledge should be a goal of EBP initiatives (Chapter 9 suggests ways to build organizational EBP infrastructure). Nurse leaders not only should support staff education initiatives that teach nurses how to read and interpret evidence, but also should themselves become familiar with desired attributes of such reviews so they can serve as credible mentors in the change process.

The challenge to the nurse is to combine the contributions of the two evidence types (research and non-research) in making patient care decisions. According to Melnyk and Fineout-Overholt (2006), no "magic bullet" or standard formula exists with which to determine how much weight should be applied to each of these factors when making patient care decisions. It is not sufficient to apply a standard rating system that grades the strength and quality of evidence without determining whether recommendations made by the best evidence are compatible with the patient's values and preferences and the clinician's expertise. Nurse leaders can best support EBP by providing clinicians with the knowledge and skills necessary to appraise quantitative and qualitative research evidence within the context of non-research evidence. Only through continuous learning can clinicians gain the confidence needed to incorporate the broad range of evidence into the more targeted care of individual patients.

Summary

This chapter describes non-research evidence, strategies for evaluating this evidence, and recommends approaches for building nurses' capacity to appraise non-research evidence to inform their practice. Non-research evidence includes summaries of evidence (clinical practice guidelines, consensus or position statements, literature reviews); organizational experience (quality improvement and financial data); expert opinion (individual commentary or opinion, case reports); community standards; clinician experience; and consumer experience. This evidence includes important information for practice decisions. For example, consumer preference is an essential element of the EBP process with increased focus on patient-centered care. In summary, while non-research evidence does not have the rigor of research evidence, it does provide important information for informed practice decisions.

References

The AGREE Research Trust. (2009). The AGREE Instrument. Retrieved from http://www.agreetrust.org/

Baharestani, M. M., & Ratliff, C. T. (2007). Pressure ulcers in neonates and children: A NPUAP white paper. *Advances in Skin & Wound Care, 20*(4), 208-220.

Benner, P. E. (2001). *From novice to expert: Excellence and power in clinical nursing practice.* (Commemorative edition). Upper Saddle River, NJ: Prentice Hall.

Birkel, R. C., Hall, L. L., Lane, T., Cohan, K., & Miller, J. (2003). Consumers and families as partners in implementing evidence-based practice. *Psychiatric Clinics of North America, 26*(4), 867-881.

Black, H. K., & Rubenstein, R. L. (2005). Direct care workers' response to dying and death in the nursing home: A case study. The Journals of Gerontology Series B: Psychological Sciences and Social Sciences, *60,* S3-S10.

Brouwers, M. C., Kho, M. E., Browman, G. P., Burgers, J. S., Cluzeau, F., Feder, G., ... Makarski, J. (2010). Development of the AGREE II, part 1: Performance, usefulness and areas for improvement. *Canadian Medical Association Journal, 182*(10), 1045-1062.

Carande-Kulis, V. G., Maciosek, M. V., Briss, P. A., Teutsch, S. M., Zaza, S., Truman, B. I., ... Fielding, J., & Task Force on Community Preventive Services. (2003). Methods for systematic reviews of economic evaluations. *American Journal of Preventive Medicine, 18*(1S), 75-91.

Carper, B. (1978). Fundamental patterns of knowing in nursing. ANS. *Advances in Nursing Science, 1*(1), 13-23.

Centers for Disease Control and Prevention (CDC). (2007). Economic evaluation of public health preparedness and response efforts. Retrieved from http://www.cdc.gov/owcd/EET/SeriesIntroduction/TOC.html

Christensen, M., & Hewitt-Taylor, J. (2006). From expert to task, expert nursing practice redefined? *Journal of Clinical Nursing, 15*(12), 1531-1539.

Community guide economic evaluation abstraction form, version 4.0. (2010). Retrieved from http://www.thecommunityguide.org/about/EconAbstraction_v5.pdf

Conn, V. S. (2004). Meta-analysis research. *Journal of Vascular Nursing, 22*(2), 51-52.

Dale, A. E. (2006). Determining guiding principles for evidence-based practice. *Nursing Standard, 20*(25), 41-46.

Dans, A. M., Dans, L., Oxman, A. D., Robinson, V., Acuin, J., Tugwell, P., ... Kang, D. (2007). Assessing equity in clinical practice guidelines. *Journal of Clinical Epidemiology, 60*(6), 540-546.

Deresinski, S., & File, T. M., Jr. (2011). Improving clinical practice guidelines—The answer is more clinical research. *Archives of Internal Medicine, 171*(15), 1402-1403.

Detsky, A. S. (2006). Sources of bias for authors of clinical practice guidelines. *Canadian Medical Association Journal, 175*(9), 1033, 1035.

Fervers, B., Burgers, J. S., Haugh, M. C., Brouwers, M., Browman, G., Cluzeau, F., & Philip, T. (2005). Predictors of high quality clinical practice guidelines: Examples in oncology. *International Journal for Quality in Health Care, 17*(2), 123-132.

Grant, M. J., & Booth, A. (2009). A typology of reviews: An analysis of 14 review types and associated methodologies. *Health Information and Libraries Journal, 26*(2), 91-108.

Hardy, S., Titchen, A., Manley, K., & McCormack, B. (2006). Re-defining nursing expertise in the United Kingdom. *Nursing Science Quarterly, 19*(3), 260-264.

Henderson, E. (2010). Sepsis mortalities cut 50% with ED changes. *ED Nursing, 13,* 93-94.

Institute for Healthcare Improvement (IHI). (2011). STate Action on Avoidable Rehospitalizations (STAAR) Initiative. Retrieved from http://www.ihi.org/offerings/Initiatives/STAAR/Pages/GetInvolved.aspx

Institute of Medicine (IOM). (1992). *Guidelines for clinical practice: From development to use.* M. J. Field & K. N. Lohr (Eds.). Washington DC: National Academy Press.

Institute of Medicine (IOM). (2001). *Crossing the quality chasm: A new health system for the 21st century.* Washington DC: National Academy Press.

Institute of Medicine (2011). *Clinical practice guidelines we can trust.* Retrieved from www.iom.edu/cpgstandards

Kazemi, D., Behan, J., & Boniauto, M. (2011). Improving teaching strategies in an undergraduate community health nursing (CHN) program: Implementation of a service-learning preceptor program. *Nurse Education Today, 31*(6), 547-52.

Kuehn, B. M. (2011). IOM sets out "gold standard" practices for creating guidelines, systematic reviews. *JAMA. 305*(18), 1846-8.

Lach, H. W. (2010) The costs and outcomes of falls: What's a nursing administrator to do? *Nursing Administration Quarterly, 34*(2), 147–155.

Lopez-Olivo, M. A., Kallen, M. A., Ortiz, Z., Skidmore, B., & Suarez-Almazor, M. E. (2008). Quality appraisal of clinical practice guidelines and consensus statements on the use of biologic agents in rheumatoid arthritis: A systematic review. *Arthritis & Rheumatism, 59*(11), 1625-1638.

Melnyk, B. M., & Fineout-Overholt, E. (2006). Consumer preferences and values as an integral key to evidence-based practice. *Nursing Administration Quarterly, 30*(2), 123-127.

Milton, C. (2007). Evidence-based practice: Ethical questions for nursing. *Nursing Science Quarterly, 20*(2), 123-126.

Morris, J., Franklin, S., & Menger, F. (2011). Returning to work with aphasia: A case study. *Aphasiology, 25*(8), 890-907.

Mosca, L., Benjamin, E., Berra, K., Bezanson, J. L., Dolor, R. J., Lloyd-Jones, D. M. ... Zhao, D. (2011). Effectiveness-based guidelines for the prevention of cardiovascular disease in women—2011 update: A guideline from the American Heart Association. *Circulation, 123*(11), 1243-62.

National Guideline Clearinghouse (NGC). (2011). Criteria for inclusion of clinical practice guidelines in NGC. Retrieved from http://www.guideline.gov/about/inclusion-criteria.aspx

Newhouse, R. P., Pettit, J. C., Poe, S., & Rocco, L. (2006). The slippery slope: Differentiating between quality improvement and research. *Journal of Nursing Administration, 36*(4), 211-219.

Polit, D. F., & Beck, C. T. (2010). *Essentials of nursing research: Appraising evidence for nursing practice.* (7th edition). Philadelphia: Wolters Kluwer|Lippincott Williams & Wilkens.

Ricketts, B. (2011). The role of simulation for learning within pre-registration nursing education — A literature review. *Nurse Education Today, 31*(7), 650-654

Shiffman, R. N., Shekelle, P., Overhage, M., Slutsky, J., Grimshaw, J., & Deshpande, A. M. (2003). Standardized reporting of clinical practice guidelines: A proposal from the conference on guideline standardization. *Annals of Internal Medicine, 139,* 493-498.

Singleton, J., & Levin, R. (2008). Strategies for Learning Evidence-Based Practice: Critically Appraising Clinical Practice Guidelines. *Journal of Nursing Education, 47*(8), 380–383.

Sise, C. B., Sise, M. J., Kelley, D. M., Walker, S. B., Calvo, R. Y., Shackford, S. R., ... Osler, T. M. (2011). Resource commitment to improve outcomes and increase value at a level I trauma center. *The Journal of Trauma: Injury, Infection, & Critical Care, 70*(3), 560-568.

Stetler, C. B., Morsi, D., Rucki, S., Broughton, S., Corrigan, B., Fitzgerald, J., ... Sheridan, E. A. (1998). Utilization-focused integrative reviews in a nursing service. *Applied Nursing Research, 11*(4), 195-206.

Weaver, C. M. (2010). Consumer-driven healthcare: What is it? *The Journal of Medical Practice Management. 25*(5), 263-265

Whittemore R. (2005). Combining evidence in nursing research: Methods and implications. *Nursing Research, 54*(1), 56-62.

Yoder-Wise, P. S. (2011). *Leading and managing in nursing* (4th ed.). St. Louis, MO: Mosby.

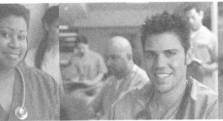
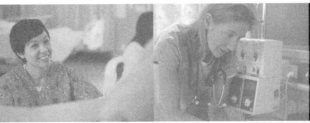

Translation

Robin P. Newhouse, PhD, RN, NEA-BC, FAAN

Kathleen White, PhD, RN, NEA-BC, FAAN

The final phase of the PET process is *translation*, which assesses the recommendations identified in the evidence phase for transferability to the desired practice setting. If appropriate, the practices are implemented, evaluated, and communicated, both within and outside the organization. Translation is the value-added step in evidence-based practice, leading to a change in nursing processes or systems and in resulting outcomes. This chapter covers the *translation* phase of PET, which includes the practice decision, implementation, and dissemination. The chapter's objectives are to

- Discuss criteria that determine recommendation implementation

- Distinguish among EBP, research, and quality improvement (QI)

- Describe the components of an action plan

- Identify steps in implementing change

- Discuss potential forums for communicating and disseminating results

Translation is the primary reason to conduct an evidence-based review. Particular attention to the planning and implementation of recommendations can improve the potential for successfully meeting the project's goals. Additionally, fully realized translation requires organizational resources and commitment. Critically appraising, rating, and grading the evidence and making practice recommendations requires one set of skills; translation requires another. Change theory, motivational theory, political savvy, organizational processes, and dynamics of power all flourish within translation.

Implementing Practice Recommendations

When you are discussing translation, the first question to consider is this: Should we implement this practice recommendation? The use of a model or framework for translation is important in answering this question and ensuring a systematic approach to the change. The JHNEBP Project Management Guide (see Appendix A) is helpful in this regard and recommends the following process:

- Determine the fit, feasibility, and appropriateness of recommendations for the translation path.

- Create an action plan and secure the support and resources necessary to carry it out.

- Implement the plan, evaluate the outcomes, and report these to stakeholders.

- Identify the next steps to continue and spread the implementation and disseminate the findings.

Additional Models for Translation

There are several other interesting frameworks specifically focused on the key elements to consider during the translation phase of an EBP project and implementation of new evidence into practice. The model developed for the Agency for Healthcare Research and Quality (AHRQ, 2002) as part of their safety initiative, includes three phases for knowledge transfer into practice.

- The first phase is *knowledge creation and distillation*. Knowledge creation is the process of research; equally important is knowledge distillation, the process of looking for evidence to improve practice and synthesizing it in a way that it can be understood by end users.

- The second phase is diffusion and dissemination. In this phase, attention is focused on identifying and developing partnerships to communicate the new evidence, to create messages about the new knowledge, and to target audiences with these messages to influence acceptance.

- The third phase is end-user adoption, implementation, and institutionalization. This phase involves interventions to translate the new evidence into practice for sustainability and routinization of the practice change (Nieva et al., 2005).

The University of Ottawa's Knowledge to Action (KTA) model uses the word *action* rather than *practice* because it is intended for a wider range of users of knowledge and not just clinicians (Graham, Tetroe, & KT Theories Research Group, 2007). The KTA process includes identifying a problem for review, adapting new knowledge to the local context, assessing barriers to use, selecting interventions to promote the knowledge, monitoring its use, evaluating the outcomes, and ensuring sustainability in practice.

The Promoting Action on Research Implementation in Health Services (PAR-IHS) model, used widely in nursing, identifies essential determinants of successful implementation of research into clinical practice. The three core elements are the nature of the *evidence*, the quality of the *context* or the environment in which the implementation will occur, and the *facilitation* strategies for translating evidence into practice (Kitson et al., 2008).

Finally, the Translation Research Model (Titler & Everett, 2001; Titler, 2010) is built on the important diffusion of innovations work by Everett Rogers (2003) and provides a framework for selecting strategies to promote adoption of evidence-based practices. According to this framework, adoption of new evidence into practice is influenced by the type and strength of the evidence, the communication or dissemination plan, the clinicians, and the characteristics of the organization.

Requirements for Successful Translation

In the past, evidence known to work has often not been implemented or has been implemented inconsistently. As the quest to improve quality of health care has increased in importance, evidence translation has achieved a higher priority. In addition, better systematic implementation strategies and frameworks have been developed to escalate the translation process.

Fully realized translation requires organizational support, human and material resources, and a commitment of individuals and interprofessional teams. Context, communication, leadership, mentoring, and evidence matter for the implementation and dissemination of new knowledge into practice. Critical to successful translation of evidence into practice are planning and active coordination by the EBP team, adherence to principles of change that guide the translation process, and careful attention to the characteristics of the organization involved (Newhouse, 2007a; White & Dudley-Brown, 2011).

Pathways to Translation

The evidence phase of the PET process ends when the team develops recommendations based on the synthesis of findings and strength of the evidence. In the JHNEBP Model, the team has four possible pathways for translating evidence into practice based on the type of available evidence:

- Strong, compelling evidence, consistent results
- Good evidence, consistent results
- Good evidence, conflicting results
- Insufficient or absent evidence

Strong, compelling evidence, consistent results. When strong, compelling evidence is available, the application to practice is quite clear, particularly if the evidence includes several level I research studies. For example, it is easy to recommend a practice change if you have three, high-quality, randomized, controlled trials with consistent results, or if there is a meta-analysis (level I) related to the question. However, this is not often the case with nursing questions.

Good evidence, consistent results. In many cases, the EBP team encounters good overall evidence yielding consistent findings across studies, but the design and quality may vary. They may have concerns about control of bias (i.e., internal and external validity); adequate comparisons; or study design and methods for which conclusions cannot be drawn. For example, the team may find only non-experimental studies without comparison groups or only descriptive correlational surveys. Or the evidence may include multiple study designs such as quasi-experimental, non-experimental, and an expert opinion. In these circumstances, and particularly in the absence of level I evidence, evaluation of the potential risks and benefits is in order before recommending a change in practice. If the benefits outweigh the risks, the EBP team should develop a pilot to test any practice change and evaluate outcomes prior to full-scale implementation.

Good evidence, conflicting results. In this situation, the overall evidence summary includes studies with conflicting findings. Such evidence is difficult to interpret. When this is the case, undertaking a practice change cannot be recommended. The EBP team may decide to review the literature periodically for new evidence to answer their question, or perhaps, to conduct their own research study.

Insufficient or absent evidence. Where little or no evidence exists in the public domain to answer the EBP question, a practice change cannot be recommended. The team may decide to search for new evidence periodically, to design their own research study, or to discontinue the project entirely.

Criteria for Successful Translation

Practice recommendations made in the evidence phase, even if based on strong evidence, cannot be implemented in all settings. The EBP team is responsible to determine the fit, feasibility, and appropriateness of recommendations for translation path. The main questions to be considered are these: Can this practice change be implemented given the current organizational infrastructure? What additional action or resources are needed? Specific criteria can be helpful to make this determination. Stetler (2001, 2010) recommends using the criteria of *substantiating evidence*, *fit of setting*, *feasibility*, and *current practice*.

When considering the overall evidence summary, the team should assess the finding's *consistency* (were results the same in the other evidence reviewed), *quality* (extent to which bias was minimized in individual studies) and *quantity* (number, sample size and power, and size of effect; Agency for Healthcare Research and Quality, 2002).

Organizational context and infrastructure, such as resources (equipment or products), change agency (linkages with people who foster change or adoption of evidence), and organizational readiness, also need to be considered (Greenhalgh, Robert, Bate, Macfarlane, & Kyriakidou, 2005). Additionally, nursing-related factors, such as nursing processes, policies, and competencies, need to be present before implementing recommendations. The following guiding questions can help to determine if the proposed recommendation adds value:

- Would this change improve clinical outcomes?
- Would this change improve patient or nurse satisfaction?
- Would this change reduce the cost of care for patients?
- Would this change improve unit operations?

Determining the feasibility of implementing EBP recommendations is very important in assessing whether they add significant value to improving a specific problem. Implementing processes with a low likelihood of success wastes valuable time and resources on efforts that produce negligible benefits.

The team should also assess the system's readiness for change, and determine strategies to overcome possible barriers to implementation. Readiness for change includes the availability of human and material resources, current processes, support from decision makers (individuals and groups), and budget implications. Implementation strategies include communication and education plans, and involvement of stakeholders and other individuals affected by the change.

Evidence-Based Practice, Research, and Quality Improvement

Although a discussion of how to conduct research to test a new procedure or product is beyond the scope of this chapter, it is important to clearly differentiate the activities of research, quality improvement (QI), and EBP (Newhouse, 2007b; Newhouse, Pettit, Rocco, & Poe, 2006). Box 8.1 provides the common definitions and an example of each. It should be noted that research requires additional organizational infrastructure, including affiliation with an Institutional Review Board (IRB), experienced mentors who can serve as principal investigators, education in human subject research, and a number of additional research competencies.

Box 8.1   Differentiating EBP, Quality Improvement, and Research

EBP

This book focuses on EBP and the Practice question, Evidence, and Translation process (PET). The PET process is used to make a decision when a significant clinical, administrative, or educational problem arises that requires a critical review of scientific and nonscientific evidence. The evidence is summarized using a rating scale; recommendations are made based on the evidence, and are implemented and evaluated. The PET process uses the organization's quality improvement (QI) program to implement recommendations and evaluate outcomes.

EBP Example: Clinical practice question: *For adult patients admitted with heart failure, what is the best education strategy for an improved smoking cessation attempt?* An evidence review is conducted using the PET process and recommendations generated. These are implemented, and evaluated using the QI process.

Quality Improvement

In QI, individuals work together for improvements within an organization's systems and processes with the intent to improve outcomes (Committee on Assessing the System for Protecting Human Research Participants, 2002). Alternatively, they may use a data-driven, systematic approach to improve care locally (Baily, Bottrell, Lynn, & Jennings, 2006). QI results are often disseminated outside the organization in the form of lessons learned, but are not generalizable beyond the organization.

QI Example: Standard measurement of compliance with smoking cessation counseling for patients with heart failure. Compliance with the smoking cessation standard is measured as present or absent for patients and is reported for improvement purposes and public information.

Research

Research is "a systematic investigation, including research development, testing, and evaluation, designed to develop or contribute to generalizable knowledge" (Department of Health and Human Services, 2005, 45 CFR 46.102[d]). Examples of research include testing changes in current practice, comparing standard care with new approaches, or evaluating new health care strategies or therapies to expand what is known (National Bioethics Advisory Commission, 2001). Research activities are intended to be generalized or applied outside an organization and require compliance with Office for Human Research Protections (OHRP) regulations, and sometimes, with the Food and Drug Administration (FDA).

Research Example: A randomized controlled design is used to test whether a new, nurse-intensive counseling session prior to discharge is more effective than standard teaching to improve smoking cessation attempts for patients who have a diagnosis of heart failure.

Creating an Action Plan for Translation

Creating an action plan provides manageable steps to implement change and assigns responsibility for carrying the project forward. The EBP team develops specific change strategies to introduce, promote, and evaluate the practice change. The action plan includes

- Development of (or a change to) a protocol, guideline, critical pathway, system, or process related to the EBP question

- Specification of a detailed timeline, assignment of team members to tasks, evaluation process, and reporting of results

- Solicitation of feedback on the action plan from organizational leadership, bedside clinicians, and other stakeholders

The action plan should be incorporated into the QI activities of the unit, department, or organization using organizational tools, processes, and reporting mechanisms. EBP teams commonly use the Model for Improvement developed by

Associates in Process Improvement (2010), which includes a process called the Plan-Do-Study-Act (PDSA) cycle. Tips for using this process and tools are available on the Institute for Healthcare Improvement (IHI) website (2011a). Steps in the model include forming the team, setting aims, establishing measures, selecting changes, implementing changes, and spreading changes (IHI, 2011a). It can be helpful to formulate the plan in a template that includes a timeline with progress columns. The Project Management Guide (see Appendix A), or a similar organizational template, can be used to monitor progress.

The action plan begins with an organizational assessment to evaluate the readiness of the organization or the context for change. Organizational infrastructure is the cornerstone of successful translation (Newhouse, 2010b). Infrastructure provides human and material resources that are fundamental in preparation for change (Greenhalgh, Robert, Bate, Macfarlane, & Kyriakidou, 2005; Newhouse, 2007a). Organizational readiness is leveraged by assessing the current state and strategically planning for building the capacity of the organization before implementation can begin.

Beyond human and material readiness, teams also need to consider organizational culture. Organizational culture refers to group-learned assumptions as the organization integrates and adapts to external forces. These assumptions become an attribute of the group and are then taught as the right way to "perceive, think, and feel in relation to problems" (Schein, 2004, p. 17). To change the culture, the team must challenge tradition, reinforce the need for evidence to drive decisions, change old patterns of behavior, and sometimes require new skills in evidence review. Additional detail and tools to assess organizational readiness and culture are available elsewhere (Newhouse, 2010a).

Steps in Implementing Change

Adoption of new knowledge theories can guide and inform effective strategies to enable a successful implementation process (Greenhalgh, Robert, Bate, Macfarlane, & Kyriakidou, 2005; Rogers, 2003). What is known about the state of current organizational change theory can be applied to EBP initiatives (Newhouse, 2007a).

Secure Support and Resources

Securing support from decision-makers is critical to implementation of recommendations. Allocation of human and material resources is dependent on the endorsement of stakeholders such as organizational leaders or committees and on collaboration with those individuals or groups affected by the recommendations. These resources should be estimated and budgeted, and an implementation plan formulated. Decision-makers may support wide implementation of the change, request a small test of the change to validate results, revise the plan or recommendations, or reject the implementation plan. Preparing for the presentation or meeting with decision-makers, involving stakeholders, and creating a comprehensive implementation plan are key steps in building organizational support.

Implement the Action Plan

After creating an action plan and securing support, implementation begins. The first step is a small test of the change, or *pilot*. The implementation plan is communicated to all team members who are affected by the change or who are caring for a patient/population affected by the change. This communication can take the form of an agenda item at a staff meeting, an inservice, direct mail, e-mail, a bulletin board, a video, and so on. Team members must know who the leader responsible for the change is and where to access needed information or supplies. Changes are then implemented and evaluated.

Evaluate Outcomes

After the change is implemented, the next step is to evaluate its impact and progress toward the desired outcome. Outcomes identified when formulating your PICO are the metrics used to evaluate the success of the change. Collaborating with the organization's QI staff is helpful during the evaluation process for guidance on the tools and the appropriate intervals to measure the change. Selecting and developing the metrics includes defining the purpose of measurement, choosing the clinical areas to evaluate, selecting the indicators, developing design specifications for the measures, and evaluating the indicators (Pronovost, Miller, Dorman, Berenholtz, & Rubin, 2001 [adapted from McGlynn, 1998]). Measures may include *process measures* (focus on steps in the system), *outcome measures* (focus on results of system performance) or *balancing measures* (focus on impact on other parts of the system; IHI, 2011b). Data collected are compared to baseline data to determine whether the change should be implemented on a wider scale. Descriptive data, such as *frequencies* or *means,* can be graphically displayed in bar, line, or run charts.

Report Outcomes to Stakeholders

After the outcome evaluation, the team should follow with a report to the appropriate committee or decision-makers. Decision-makers can be a committee, such as a research or quality improvement committee, or organizational leaders. The report should be a succinct communication, in executive summary format, consistent with organizational templates. Box 8.2 provides an example of an executive summary framed in the PET template.

Box 8.2   Example of Template for Executive Summary Using PET

Problem

There is an increase in the incidence of postoperative pressure ulcers. When patients are positioned in the operating room, the team uses multiple positioning aids, and no standard for positioning based on the type of surgery exists.

Practice Question

What are the most effective interventions to prevent skin pressure in adult patients undergoing surgery?

Evidence

CINAHL and PubMed were searched using the key words *perioperative* or *surgery,* AND *positioning,* AND *pressure ulcers;* 18 sources of evidence were reviewed.

Recommendations

1. Identify a team from the perioperative and inpatient areas to develop a comprehensive pressure ulcer prevention protocol that includes all perioperative phases (preoperatively through discharge).

2. The Nurse Manager of the OR will evaluate the use of current pressure-relieving devices for patients at risk and report current practices and compliance to the nursing Quality Improvement Committee.

3. The OR Quality Improvement committee will evaluate gel and alternating pressure mattresses in the OR and recommend changes if indicated to the Products Committee and the OR Procedure Committee.

4. The OR Procedure Committee will review and standardize OR positioning protocols.

5. The OR Evidence-based Practice Committee will develop a risk assessment/screening tool for patients undergoing surgery.

Identify Next Steps

After successful implementation and favorable evaluation of recommendations, and with support from decision-makers, changes are implemented on a wider scale, if appropriate. The team reviews the process and results and considers the next steps. Organization-wide, or additional unit implementation requires a modified action plan and possibly redesignation of responsibilities to an individual, team, or committee. Considerations for the new team can include: a new question that emerges from the process, additional training or education for colleagues involved in the process change, and suggestions for new measures or tools for the evaluation. The recommendations are then implemented and evaluated.

Disseminate Findings

The level of communication regarding the findings and dissemination of information is a factor of the problem's scope. Evidence-based project outcomes are communicated internally to all members involved in the care of the patient or population affected by the practice changes. This communication can take the form of internal meetings, committees or conferences, or publications in newsletters, or the intranet.

Additionally, it may be appropriate to present results at professional conferences or in suitable EBP publications, sharing lessons learned, what worked, what did not, the resulting clinical and fiscal outcomes, and so on. Methods of external dissemination may also include podium or poster presentations, publication in electronic media, or publications in journals whose focus is quality improvement.

Specific guidance on how to develop abstracts, presentations, and publications is available (Krenzischek & Newhouse, 2005). Presentations at local, national, and international professional organizations or university conferences are an excellent way to gain presentation experience. See Table 8.1 for links to general and specialty organization websites. Search each website for appropriate conferences, dates, and locations and communicate the opportunity via group e-mail, mail, or the organization's intranet. Announcements of upcoming conferences generally include information about calls for abstracts; each abstract has specific instructions for content, length, and responsibilities.

Table 8.1   Websites for Potential Conferences to Present EBP Projects

Organization	Website
Sigma Theta Tau International	www.nursingsociety.org
American Nurses Association General Nursing Practice Links	www.nursingworld.org
American Nurses Association Specialty Nursing Practice Links	www.nursingworld.org
American Nurses Credentialing Center National Magnet Conference	www.nursecredentialing.org/

Many professional nursing and multidisciplinary journals and newsletters publish manuscripts about EBP projects. Author guidelines are usually available via the Internet for review. *Worldviews on Evidence-Based Nursing* focuses specifically on EBP and is an excellent resource for a potential publication.

Summary

Translation is the outcome of the PET process. The PET process is linear, but many steps in the process can generate new questions, recommendations, or actions. The organizational infrastructure needed to foster translation includes budgetary support, human and material resources, and the commitment of individuals, stakeholders, and interprofessional teams. Translation is the essence of the evidence-based practice process and the cornerstone of best practice. Translation of recommendations requires organizational skills, project management, and leaders with a high level of influence and tenacity—the perfect job for nurses.

References

Agency for Healthcare Research and Quality. (2002). *Systems to rate the strength of scientific evidence. Summary, Evidence report/Technology assessment: Number 47* (Rep. No. 02-E015). Rockville, MD. Available at http://archive.ahrq.gov/clinic/epcsums/strengthsum.htm

Associates in Process Improvement. (2010). Model for Improvement. Available at http://www.apiweb.org/API_home_page.htm

Baily, M. A., Bottrell, M., Lynn, J., & Jennings, B. (2006). *The ethics of using QI methods to improve health care quality and safety: A Hastings Center special report.* Garrison, New York: The Hastings Center.

Committee on Assessing the System for Protecting Human Research Participants. (2002). *Responsible research: A systems approach to protecting research participants.* Washington, DC: The National Academies Press.

Department of Health and Human Services. (2005). Code of Federal Regulations TITLE 45 PUBLIC WELFARE PART 46 PROTECTION OF HUMAN SUBJECTS. Department of Health and Human Services. Available at http://www.hhs.gov/ohrp/policy/ohrpregulations.pdf

Graham, I., Tetroe, J., and the KT Theories Research Group. (2007). Some theoretical underpinnings of knowledge translation. *Academic Emergency Medicine, 14*(11), 936-941.

Greenhalgh, T., Robert, G., Bate, P., Macfarlane, A., & Kyriakidou, O. (2005). *Diffusion of innovations in health service organizations: A systematic literature review.* Massachusetts: Blackwell Publishing Ltd.

Institute for Healthcare Improvement (IHI). (2011a). How to improve. Retrieved from http://www.ihi.org/knowledge/Pages/HowtoImprove/default.aspx

Institute for Healthcare Improvement (IHI). (2011b). Science of improvement: Establishing measures. Retrieved from http://www.ihi.org/knowledge/Pages/HowtoImprove/ScienceofImprovementEstablishingMeasures.aspx

Kitson, A., Rycroft-Malone, J., Harvey, G., McCormack, B., Seers, K., & Titchen, A. (2008). Evaluating the successful implementation of evidence into practice using the PARiHS framework: Theoretical and practical challenges. *Implementation Science*, 3(1). Retrieved from http://www.implementationscience.com/content/pdf/1748-5908-3-1.pdf

Krenzischek, D. A., & Newhouse, R. (2005). Dissemination of findings. In R. Newhouse & S. Poe (Eds.), *Measuring Patient Safety* (pp. 67-78). Boston: Jones and Bartlett Publishers.

McGlynn, E. A. (1998). Choosing and evaluating clinical performance measures. *Joint Commission Journal of Quality Improvement*, 24(9): 470-479.

National Bioethics Advisory Commission. (2001). *Ethical and policy issues in research involving human participants*. Bethesda, MD: Author.

Newhouse, R. P. (2007a). Creating infrastructure supportive of evidence-based nursing practice: Leadership strategies. *Worldviews on Evidence-Based Nursing, 4*(1), 21-29.

Newhouse, R. P. (2007b). Diffusing confusion among evidence-based practice, quality improvement, and research. *Journal of Nursing Administration, 37*(10), 432-435.

Newhouse, R. P. (2010a). Instruments to assess organizational readiness for evidence-based practice. *Journal of Nursing Administration*, 40(10), 404-407.

Newhouse, R. P. (2010b). Establishing organizational infrastructure. In S. S. Poe and K. M. White (Eds.), *Johns Hopkins Nursing Evidence-Based Practice Implementation and Translation* (pp. 55-72). Sigma Theta Tau International: Indianapolis, IN.

Newhouse, R. P., Pettit, J. C., Poe, S., & Rocco, L. (2006). The slippery slope: Differentiating between quality improvement and research. *Journal of Nursing Administration, 36*(4), 211-219.

Nieva, V. F., Murphy, R., Ridley, N., Donaldson, N., Combes, J., Mitchell, P., ... Carpenter, D. (2005). From science to service: A framework for the transfer of patient safety research into practice. In K. Henriksen, J. B. Battles, E. S. Marks et al. (Eds.), *Advances in patient safety: From research to implementation (Volume 2: Concepts and methodology)*. Rockville, MD: Agency for Healthcare Research and Quality (US).

Pronovost, P. J., Miller, M. R., Dorman, T., Berenholtz, S. M., & Rubin, H. (2001). Developing and implementing measures of quality of care in the intensive care unit. *Current Opinions in Critical Care*, 7(4), 297-303.

Rogers, E. M. (2003). *Diffusions of innovations* (5th ed.). New York: The Free Press.

Schein, E. H. (2004). *Organizational culture and leadership* (3rd ed.). San Francisco: Jossey-Bass.

Stetler, C. B. (2001). Updating the Stetler Model of research utilization to facilitate evidence-based practice. *Nursing Outlook, 49*(6), 272-279.

Stetler, C. B. (2010). Stetler model. In J. Rycroft-Malone & T. Bucknall (Eds.), *Evidence-based practice series. Models and frameworks for implementing evidence-based practice: Linking evidence to action*. Oxford: Wiley-Blackwell.

Titler, M. G., & Everett, L. Q. (2001). Translating research into practice: Considerations for critical care investigators. *Critical Care Nursing Clinics of North America*, 13(4), 587-604.

Titler, M. G. (2010). Translation science and context. *Research and Theory in Nursing Practice* 24(1), 35-55.

White, K. M., & Dudley-Brown, S. (2011). *Translation of evidence into nursing and health care practice.* New York: Springer Publishing

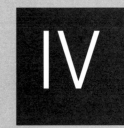

IV

Infrastructure

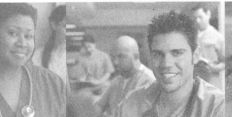
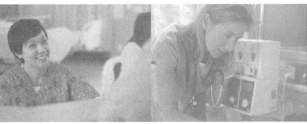

9

Creating a Supportive Evidence-Based Practice Environment

Kathleen White, PhD, RN, NEA-BC, FAAN
Deborah Dang, PhD, RN, NEA, BC

Why be concerned about creating a supportive environment for evidence-based practice (EBP)? The most obvious answer is that new evidence is continually surfacing in nursing and medical environments. Practitioners must incorporate the tremendous increase in the generation of new knowledge into their daily routine for their practice to be evidence-based, yet there is a well-documented delay in implementing new knowledge into practice environments. Balas & Boren (2000) cited 17 years as the average time from generation of new evidence to implementation of that evidence into practice. Additionally, for health care professionals to keep up with journals relevant to practice, every practitioner would need to read 17 articles per day, 365 days per year (Balas & Boren, 2000).

Our dynamic and competitive health care environment requires health care practitioners who are accountable to provide efficient and effective care. This environment also mandates continuous improvement in care processes and outcomes. Health care, provided within the structure of a system or organization, can either facilitate or inhibit the uptake of evidence. EBP requires the creation of an environment that fosters lifelong learning to increase the use of evidence in practice.

Because of the emphasis on quality and safety, many health care organizations have created strategic initiatives for EBP. Current national pay-for-performance initiatives, both voluntary and mandatory, provide reimbursement to hospitals and practitioners for implementing health care practices supported with evidence. Consumer pressure and increased patient expectations lend an even greater emphasis on this need for true evidence-based practice. However, McGlynn et al. (2003), in an often-cited study, reported that Americans receive only about 50% of the health care recommended by evidence. Therefore, even with an increased emphasis on EBP, the majority of hospitals and practitioners are not implementing the available evidence and guidelines for care in their practices. This suggests an even greater imperative for building infrastructure that not only supports EBP but also infuses it into practice environments.

Over the last 10 years, three Institute of Medicine (IOM) reports have called for health care professionals to focus on evidence-based practice. In 2001, *Crossing the Quality Chasm: A New Health System for the 21st Century*, called for the health care system to adopt six aims for improvement and ten principles for redesign, citing "the nation's health care delivery system has fallen far short in its ability to translate knowledge into practice and to apply new technology safely and appropriately" (p. 3). The report also recommended that health care decision-making be evidence-based to ensure patients receive care based on the best scientific evidence available and that this evidence be transparent to patients and their families to assist them in making informed decisions. The second report, *Health Professions Education: A Bridge to Quality* (2003), described five key competencies for health professionals: delivering patient-centered care, working as part of interprofessional teams, focusing on quality improvement, using information technology, and practicing evidence-based medicine. The last IOM report, *The Future of Nursing: Leading Change, Advancing Health* (2011), focused on the need to expand opportunities for nurses to collaborate with physicians and other health care team members to conduct research and to redesign and improve both practice environments and health systems to deliver quality health care. For this to happen, the report urges nursing education to ensure nurses achieve competency in leadership, health policy, systems improvement, teamwork and collaboration, and research and evidence-based practice.

The American Nurses Association revised the *Nursing: Scope and Standards for Practice* in 2010, making a substantive change to the "Research" standard by renaming it "Evidence-based Practice and Research." The new standard of professional performance requires that the "registered nurse integrates evidence and research findings into practice" (p. 51). The competencies are very specific and hold the registered nurse accountable to

- Utilize current evidence-based nursing knowledge, including research findings to guide practice

- Incorporate evidence when initiating changes in nursing practice

- Participate, as appropriate to education level and position, in the formulation of evidence-based practice through research

- Share personal or third-party research findings with colleagues and peers (ANA, 2010)

Other substantive changes throughout the standards emphasize the imperative for evidence in nursing practice and create a significantly stronger role for nurses to promote an EBP environment and advocate for resources to support research (ANA, 2010).

A new type of health care worker exists today, one educated to think critically and not simply accept the status quo. Generation Y, also known as Millenniums, and generation Z (http://www.socialmarketing.org/) nurses question current nursing practices, and "We've always done it that way" is no longer a good enough answer. They want evidence that what they are doing in the workplace is efficient and effective. These nurses are pushing the profession away from doing things because of tradition and past practices if those ways are unsupported by evidence. This push requires that evidence support all clinical, educational, and administrative decision-making.

This compelling need for EBP in our health care environments requires proper planning, development, and commitment. This chapter:

- Discusses how to choose an EBP model for use in the organization

- Explores how to create and facilitate a supportive EBP environment

- Describes how to overcome common implementation barriers

- Discusses how to sustain the change

Choosing an EBP Model

A standardized framework for EBP inquiry in the organization is needed to implement best practices both clinically and administratively, to identify and improve cost components of care, to foster outcomes improvement, and to ensure success of the EBP initiative.

Careful evaluation of any EBP model or framework being reviewed for adoption should consider

- Fit and feasibility of the model with the vision, mission, philosophy, and values of the organization and the department of nursing

- Educational background, leadership, experience, and practice needs of the nursing staff

- Presence of any partnerships for the EBP initiative, such as a school of nursing or collaboration with other professions, such as medicine, pharmacy, nutrition

- Culture and environment of the organization

- Availability and access to sources of evidence internal or external to the organization

The leadership team should appoint a group to champion the EBP process and review models using the points above and other agreed-upon criteria. Criteria for model review may include identifying strengths and weaknesses, evaluating assumptions, verifying ease of use, ensuring applicability for all clinical situations, reviewing examples of use and dissemination, and securing recommendations of other users.

Creating and Facilitating a Supportive EBP Environment

To move the evidence-based practice initiative forward, the organization's leadership must ensure that the appropriate infrastructure is available and supported. This organizational infrastructure consists of human and material resources and a receptive culture. Key assumptions regarding evidence-based nursing practice include the following:

- Nursing is both a science and an applied profession.
- Knowledge is important to professional practice, and there are limits to knowledge that must be identified.
- Not all evidence is created equal, and there is a need to use the best available evidence.
- Evidence-based practice contributes to improved outcomes. (Newhouse, 2007).

Successful infusion of evidence-based practice throughout the organization must focus on three key strategies: *establish the culture, build capacity,* and *ensure sustainability.*

Establishing the Organizational Culture

Establishing a culture of practice based on evidence is a leadership-driven change that fundamentally challenges commonly held beliefs about the practice of nursing. This transformational change in culture typically occurs over a period of 3–5 years. During this time, EBP is embedded into the values, norms, and structure of the department of nursing and caregiving units through a planned and systematic approach.

Schein (2004) defines organizational culture as "patterns of shared basic assumptions that were learned by a group as it solved its problems of external adaption and internal integration, that has worked well enough … to be taught to new members as the correct way to perceive, think, feel in relationship to these problems" (p. 17).

Thus, culture, a potent force operating below the surface, guides, constrains, and/or stabilizes the behavior of group members through shared group norms (Schein, 2004). Although organizations develop distinct cultures, subcultures also operate at the unit or team level and create a context for practice. Embedding a culture based on practice requires that nurse leaders at all levels explicitly challenge tradition, set expectations, and role model the use of evidence as the basis for decisions and hold all level of staff accountable for these behaviors.

The visible and tangible work of establishing a culture supportive of EBP requires revisiting the philosophy of nursing, developing a strategic plan, assuring leaders are committed, identifying and exploiting the use of mentors and informal leaders, and overcoming barriers.

Reviewing the Nursing Philosophy

A tangible way to signal a change to a culture of evidence-based practice and lay the foundation for leadership commitment is to review and revise the philosophy for the department of nursing. This statement should include several key points. First, the philosophy should speak to the spirit of inquiry and the lifelong learning necessary for evidence-based practice. Second, it should address a work environment that demands and supports the nurses' accountability for practice and decision-making. Finally, the philosophy needs to include the goal of improving patient care outcomes through evidence-based clinical and administrative decision-making. See Table 9.1 for an example of the Philosophy Statement for The Johns Hopkins Hospital department of nursing. At The Johns Hopkins Hospital, the vice president of nursing and the directors wanted to ensure that the revisions in the philosophy resonated with and had meaning for the staff. After they revised the document, they hosted an open forum with staff selected from all levels in the nursing department to provide input and feedback on the philosophy. This process highlighted the importance of this change, communicated leader commitment to EBP and the part that staff would have in this change and transition.

Table 9.1   Philosophy of The Johns Hopkins Hospital Department of Nursing

At The Johns Hopkins Hospital, we integrate the science of nursing, clinical knowledge, nursing judgment, and passionate commitment to quality care with the art of nursing, honoring patients' trust that they will be cared for with integrity and compassion.

In our practice...

> we are experts in the specialized treatment of illnesses;
>
> we pursue quality outcomes, advocating in the best interest of our patients;
>
> we embrace the responsibility of autonomous practice and commit to a collaborative approach to patient care;
>
> we seek, appraise, and incorporate the best evidence to support our practice;
>
> we master the application of health care technology;
>
> we pursue excellence, creativity, and innovation.

On behalf of patients and families...

> we pledge compassionate care throughout a patient's illness to recovery, discharge, or end of life;
>
> we use our skills to diagnose health concerns, intervene promptly, and monitor efficacy of treatment;
>
> we position ourselves as sentinels of safety and advocates for quality care;
>
> we honor individual uniqueness, embrace diversity, treat holistically.

As professionals...

> we bring intellectual rigor, ethical conduct, and emotional competence to our practice;
>
> we cultivate personal leadership and professional growth;
>
> we take the lead in our organization to improve patient care;
>
> we celebrate the talents of nurse colleagues, valuing positive relationships, shared governance, and mutual accountability;
>
> we advance our profession locally, nationally, and internationally;
>
> we respect the diversity of persons, of disciplines, and of communities with whom we interact.

We treasure our heritage, celebrate our present, and engage the future.

We stand in the forefront of healthcare and nursing practice.

We stand for patients.

Developing a Strategic Plan

Supportive and committed executive-level leadership, including the chief nurse executive (CNE), must be involved in the creation and development of an evidence-based practice environment. To operationalize the philosophy statement and build capacity for implementation of EBP, the organization's leaders must develop a strategic plan to identify goals and objectives, time frames, responsibilities, and an evaluation process. The plan also requires a commitment to allocate adequate resources to the EBP initiative, including people, time, money, education, and mentoring. As a strategic goal, evidence-based practice should be implemented at all levels of the organization. As the initiative rolls out, leaders need to check the pulse of the organization and be prepared to modify the strategy as necessary. To enable the process, they should identify potential barriers to implementation, have a plan to reduce or remove them, and support the project directors and change champions in every way possible. Figure 9.1 outlines the essential elements of a strategic plan for initial implementation of EBP. As EBP develops over time, the content of the strategic plan should reflect the maturation of the program.

The support and visibility of the CNE is paramount. The staff must see the CNE as a leader with a goal of infusing, building, and sustaining an evidence-based practice environment.

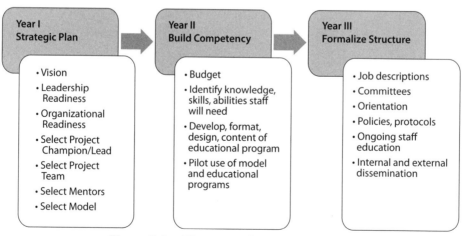

Figure 9.1   Elements of a strategic plan.

The organization's leadership can support EBP efforts best by modeling the practice and ensuring all administrative decision-making is evidence-based. For example, if the organization's leaders ask middle managers for evidence (both organizational data and the best available research and non-research evidence) to support important decisions in their areas of responsibility, it is more likely that staff at all levels will also question and require evidence for their practice decisions. Additionally, all organizational and department of nursing clinical and administrative standards (policies, protocols, and procedures) need to be evidence-based and have source citations on the standards if a need to retrieve the reference arises. For example, at The Johns Hopkins Hospital, the infection control department implemented a policy regarding the use of artificial fingernails. Because Nurse Managers (NM) were challenged with how to hold staff accountable for this change in policy, nursing leaders convened a group of NMs to conduct an EBP project on this topic. As a result, NMs were now armed with the best evidence on the risks associated with use of artificial nails and had direct experience with the EBP process and how it can strengthen administrative practice. With such leadership examples and activities, verbal and non-verbal EBP language becomes assimilated into everyday activities and establishes an evidence-based culture.

Finally, the CNE can further model support for EBP by actually participating in EBP change activities. For example, if the plan is to offer EBP education to the management group, the CNE can attend and introduce the session by discussing the organization's vision of EBP. The CNE's presence demonstrates the leadership's commitment to EBP and its value to the organization. Participating gives the CNE an appreciation for the process, including the time and resource commitment necessary for the organization to move toward an evidence-based practice.

Ensuring Committed Organizational Leadership

When leaders are actively involved and frequently consulted, the success of implementation, sustainability, and a stable infrastructure are more likely. When leaders are not engaged, the change and transition process is more reactive than proactive, and the infrastructure and sustainability over time is less certain.

Greenhalgh, Robert, Macfarlane, Bate, & Kyriakidou (2004) describe three styles for managing change and adoption of an innovation such as EBP.

- The first are leaders that "let it happen," communicating a passive style where, for example, small pockets of staff may self-organize to explore and create their own process for doing EBP.

- Leaders "help it happen" when a formal group such as advanced practice nurses, acting as change champions, have invested in and defined an approach to evidence-based practice and have to negotiate for support and resources to implement it. Still, the leader is being pulled into the process by change rather than leading it.

- The "make it happen approach" is intentional, systematic, planned and managed by, and fully engages all nurse leaders in the process, thereby ensuring adoption, spread, and sustainability.

Identifying and Developing Mentors and Informal Leaders

Mentors and change champions have a key role in assimilation of EBP into the organizational culture. They provide a safe and supportive environment for staff to move out of their comfort zone as they learn new skills and competencies. Informal leaders influence the staff at the unit or departmental level. The presence and influence of both roles is a key attribute for sustainability and building capacity within staff. Because EBP is a leadership-driven change, leaders should identify and involve both formal and informal leaders early and often in creating the change and transition strategies so they can serve as advocates rather than opponents for the change and role model its use in practice.

Leadership must identify and select mentors with care, choosing them from across the organization—different professionals, levels, and specialties. Consider who within the organization has the knowledge and skills to move an EBP initiative forward, can offer the best support, and has the most at stake to see that EBP is successful. Building the skills and knowledge of mentors should take into account such questions as, "How will the mentors be trained? Who will provide the initial training? How and by whom will they be supported after their training is complete?" As the activities to build an EBP environment increase, the leadership needs to diffuse education and mentoring activities throughout the nursing staff. The key to success is to increase buy-in by involving as many staff as possible to champion the EBP process by focusing on a problem that is important to them.

You can develop mentors in many ways. Initially, if the organization has not yet developed experts within its staff, it can find mentors through collaborative opportunities outside of the organization, such as partnerships with schools of nursing or consultation with organizations and experts who have developed models. After internal expertise is established, the implementation of EBP throughout the organization results in a self-generating mechanism for developing mentors. For example, members of committees who participate in EBP projects guided by a mentor quickly become mentors to other staff, committees, or groups who are engaged in EBP work. EBP fellowships are another way to develop mentors where the fellow gains skills to lead and consult with staff groups within their home department or throughout the organization.

Evidence indicates that nurses, when facing a clinical concern, prefer asking a colleague rather than searching a journal, book, or the internet for the answer (Pravikoff, Tanner, & Pierce, 2005). Colleagues sought out are often informal leaders, and evidence indicates that these informal leaders—opinion leaders and change champions—are effective in changing behaviors of teams if used in combination with education and performance feedback (Titler, 2008). Formal leaders differ from informal leaders in that formal leaders have position power; whereas informal leaders' power is derived from their status, expertise, and opinions within a group.

Opinion leaders are the "go-to" people with wide spheres of influence who peers would send to represent them, and they are viewed as "respected source[s] of influence, considered by peers as technically competent, are trusted to judge the fit between innovation (EBP) and the local [unit] situation … opinion leaders use of innovation [EBP] influences peers and alters group norms" (Titler, 2008, p. 1–118). Change champions have a similar impact, but they differ in that, although they practice on the unit, they are not part of the unit staff. They circulate information, encourage peers to adopt the innovation, orient staff to innovations, and are persistent and passionate about the innovation (Titler, 2008).

The identification of champions can occur at two levels. The first is at the organizational level. At The Johns Hopkins Hospital, nursing leaders have successfully used clinical leadership roles such as clinical nurse specialists, wound care, or safety nurse specialists as change champions. The second group of champions is at the departmental level and includes departmental nursing committee members who are expert clinicians whom the staff see as role models for professional practice and who can hold staff accountable. They are nurses committed to clinical inquiry and, many times, are initially identified because of their interest in the topic or issue for an EBP project, or are skillful collaborators and team players.

The critical role of mentor and informal leaders in facilitating EBP and translating the evidence into practice has been the focus of significant work (Dearholt, White, Newhouse, Pugh, & Poe, 2008; Titler, 2008). The nursing literature supports that mentoring and support are needed throughout the EBP process to help nurses be successful and to promote excellence (Block, Claffey, Korow, & McCaffrey, 2005; Carroll, 2004; Owens & Patton, 2003).

The Johns Hopkins Nursing Experience

After the JHNEBP Model was developed and ready for testing, the first group to receive education and training was the post-anesthesia care unit (PACU) staff. They were chosen for three reasons: the nurse manager was committed to EBP, the PACU had a well-established professional practice with expectations of staff nurse involvement in unit activities, and nurses had two hours of protected time scheduled each week which could be used for the training. The PACU staff proposed to examine a priority administrative and clinical practice issue related to cost, volume, satisfaction, and throughput. The question generated by the staff was, "Should ambulatory adults void before being discharged from the PACU?"

The EBP process began with education classes held in short weekly or biweekly sessions. Each week, the PACU staff was asked to evaluate the education, the model, and their satisfaction with the process. They were asked the following questions:

- Is the model clear, usable, adequate, and feasible?
- Is the staff satisfied with the evidence-based process?
- Is the staff satisfied with the outcome of the process?

The results demonstrated significant differences across time in the nurses' perceptions of the adequacy of the EBP resources, the feasibility of the process, and their satisfaction with the process and outcome. Figure 9.2 describes the mean changes in evaluation responses across time. After the initial training, nurses began the process with positive perceptions; these dropped significantly in all three areas when they began to use the model to search and evaluate evidence independently. At the end of five education sessions, the nurses' perceptions of the adequacy of EBP resources, the feasibility of the process, and their satisfaction with the process and outcome, returned to levels higher than their initial ratings.

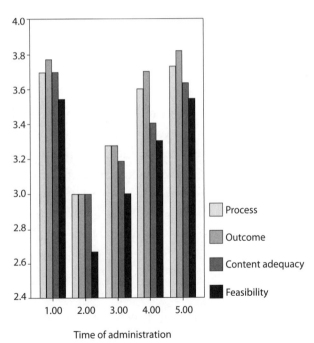

Figure 9.2   Nurse evaluation of pilot implementation of the JHNEBP Model

These results support the need for mentorship during the EBP process as nurses learn new skills, including the research and evidence appraisal work (Newhouse, Poe, Dearholt, Pugh, & White, 2005). At the end of the pilot, the EBP leadership team concluded that staff nurses can effectively use the JHNEBP Model with the help of knowledgeable mentors and that implementation of a practical EBP model is necessary to translate research into practice. The evaluation also included qualitative responses that showed enthusiasm for the EBP process and a renewed sense of professionalism and accomplishment among the nurses. Indicators of success of an environment supportive of nursing inquiry included the following:

- Staff has access to nursing reference books and the Internet on the patient care unit

- Journals are available in hard copy or online

- A medical/nursing library is available

- Knowledgeable library personnel are available to support staff and assist with evidence searches

- Other resources for inquiry and EBP are available

Estabrooks (1998) surveyed staff nurses about their use of various sources of knowledge. She found that the sources used most often by nurses were their own experiences, other workplace sources, physicians' intuition, and practices that have worked for years. Nurses ranked literature, texts, or journals in the bottom five of all sources accessed for information. Pravikoff, Tanner, and Pierce (2005) studied EBP readiness among nurses and found 61% of nurses needed to look up clinical information at least once per week. However, 67% of nurses always or frequently sought information from a colleague instead of a reference text, and 83% rarely or never sought a librarian's assistance. If an organization provides resources for practice inquiry and creates an expectation of their use, EBP can flourish. Those who do not provide such resources must address this critical need.

Overcoming Barriers

One of the ongoing responsibilities of leadership is to identify and develop a plan to overcome barriers to the implementation and maintenance of an EBP environment. This responsibility cannot be taken lightly and must be a part of the implementation plan.

Those involved in EBP have repeatedly cited *time constraints* as a barrier that prevents implementation of EBP and the continued use of an investigative model for practice. Providing clinical release time to staff participating in an EBP project is essential. Experience shows that staff need time to think about and discuss the EBP project; to read the latest evidence; and to appraise the level, strength, and quality of that evidence. Reading research and critiquing evidence is challenging and demanding work for most nurses and requires blocks of time set aside for effective work. It cannot be done in stolen moments away from the patients or in brief, 15-minute intervals. Nurses need uninterrupted time away from the clinical unit.

A *lack of supportive leadership* for EBP is another major barrier to the creation and maintenance of an EBP environment. Leadership can be facilitated through the vision, mission, philosophy, and strategic plan. The top leaders must incorporate EBP into their roles and normative behavior. In order to create a culture of organizational support for EBP, the day-to-day language must be consistent with using evidence and be a part of the organizational values. That is, leaders must *talk-the-talk*—making a point to ask, "Where is the evidence?" Leaders must also *walk-the-talk*, demonstrating a regard for evidence on a daily basis in their actions and behaviors. Does the organization value science and research and hold its staff accountable for using the best evidence in practice and clinical decision-making? Do leaders question whether routine decisions are made using the best possible data/evidence or using experience or history, financial restrictions, or even emotion? Do leaders themselves use the best evidence available for administrative decision-making? This can easily be seen if one looks at the titles for administrative staff within the organization. Is there a director or department for research or quality improvement? If there is, where are these individuals on the organizational chart? To whom do they report? Are these roles centralized or decentralized in the organizational structure?

A *lack of organizational infrastructure* to support EBP is another significant barrier. Resources, in terms of people, money, and time, need to be negotiated and allocated to support the initiative. Staff must be able to access library resources, computers, and current evidence in online database resources. Experts, such as the champions and mentors, must also be part of the available infrastructure.

Nurses themselves can be a significant barrier to implementing EBP. They often lack the skills, knowledge, and confidence to read results of research studies and translate them into practice. Some nurses also may resist EBP through negative attitudes and skepticism toward research. In some organizations, nurses may feel they have limited authority to make or change practice decisions and are skeptical that anything can result from the pursuit of evidence. Another potential barrier is the relationships of staff nurses with other nurses in the organizational hierarchy, such as clinical nurse specialists, and with physicians and other professional staff.

Barriers that come from nurses are best dealt with through prevention and planning to assess and identify staff needs. The EBP leaders, champions, and mentors can support the staff throughout the EBP process to incorporate the changes into practice. Professionals need to value each others' contribution to patient care and clinical decision-making. If the input of all staff, especially that of nurses, is not valued, a lack of interest and confidence in participating in an EBP initiative is the result.

Lack of communication is a common barrier to implementation of any change, but is particularly detrimental to EBP initiatives. This barrier can be overcome by using the strategies in the design of a communication plan for an EBP initiative. As the staff develops EBP and approaches the clinical environment with critical thinking, they want to know that what they are doing is valued. The staff expects leaders to be responsive and open to their concerns or questions as the change is implemented. Staff will take ownership of the change if they sense their leaders are partners in the change process.

A final barrier is *lack of incentives,* or rewards, in the organization for support of an EBP environment. Some think that staff should not have to be rewarded for doing their job. Leaders should consider, however, whether the organization's system includes incentives or disincentives and whether an accountability-based environment exists. Establishing an EBP environment and continuing EBP project work is challenging and requires a level of commitment on the part of all involved. Incentives can be dealt with in several areas already discussed: communication, education and mentoring, job descriptions, and evaluation tools. The leadership team should understand the need for such incentives and plan for recognition and rewards that are a part of the EBP implementation process. These are crucial discussion points during the planning, implementation, and maintenance of the change.

Leading Change and Managing Transition

A key factor for success when undergoing a culture change is that nurse leaders and those assigned to implement the change understand the difference between change and transition (see Table 9.2) and how to *lead* change and *manage* transitions (Bridges, 2009); this understanding provides insights on how to overcome the barriers previously discussed.

Table 9.2   Definitions of Change and Transition

Change	An event that starts, stops, and occurs external to us.
Transition	An emotional or psychological process that goes on inside of the hearts and minds of staff as they come to grips with the new way of doing things.

Change is an event that has a clear and tangible start and stopping point. For example, a staff-lead EBP project finds that patients and families prefer clinical staff to wear color-coded scrubwear to distinguish among different team members. Based on this evidence, a decision is made to change to standard colors for scrubwear for all clinical staff. This is change—it begins with selecting colors for clinicians and ends when staff begin wearing the new scrubs. *Transition*, on the other hand, involves letting go of something familiar which generates a feeling of loss. When staff are labeled "resistant to change," it is really the transition that they are resisting—the emotional process of "letting go" of something familiar, valued, treasured. Though change can take place in a short time period, the time trajectory for transitions is different for each person and is defined by where they are at any given moment. So, to understand why some staff may resist change, leaders of the change have to understand what staff will have to let go of if a recommendation is made to standardize scrubwear.

The amount of planning for change and transitions is directly related to the scope and complexity of the change and the amount of spread. Some changes may be a simple, straightforward communication or fast-facts education on a device, such as switching from use of a flutter valve to an incentive spirometer on a post-operative surgical unit. Or it can be complex, multifaceted, and hospital-wide, such as implementation of a nurse-managed heparin protocol that impacts nurse and physician responsibilities and workflow across the hospital. In either situation, knowing the difference between change and transition is important to success.

Strategies for Managing Transitions

Strategies for managing change are concrete and are guided by tactical plans such as those outlined in Appendix A, Project Management Guide. However, when change activities spark resistance, it is a clue that staff are dealing with transition—the human side of the change. Resistance to change is how feelings of loss are manifested, and these are not always concrete. Losses may be related to attitudes, expectations, assumptions—all of which make up staff comfort zones and provide them with a sense of routine and familiarity in what they do every day.

One way to head off resistance is to talk with staff about what they feel they stand to lose in doing things a new way—in other words, assess their losses. Another strategy to help staff move through the transition is to describe the change in as much detail as possible, being specific so staff can form a clear picture of where they are going, why, and what part they play. In assessing loss, leaders need to think of individuals and groups that will be affected by the change both directly and downstream of the practice or process that is being changed. Because transitions are a subjective experience, not all staff is going to perceive and express the same losses. Examples of the range of losses include competence, routines, relationships, status, power, meaning to their work, turf, group membership, and personal identity (Bridges, 2009). Specific strategies to address these transitions include

- Talking with staff openly to understand their perceptions of what is ending. Frontline clinicians have enormous wisdom and what they see as problems with the change should be respected and tapped into by valuing rather than judging their dissent. Do this simply, directly, and with empathy; for example, "I see your hesitation in supporting the new scrubwear decision. Help me understand why." In the end, staff are likely to move through the transition more quickly if given the chance to talk openly about their losses.

- Because culture is local, *how* the change is implemented needs to be tailored to the context of the caregiving unit where staff work; staff need to own this locally. This is one reason why informal leaders and change champions are so important.

- Clarify what is staying the same to minimize overgeneralization and overreaction to the change.

- After acknowledging the loss, honor the past for what has been accomplished. Present the change as something that builds on this past. One way to do this is with symbolic events or rituals that can be powerful markers of honoring the past. For example, staff may create a quilt or collage of pieces or patterns of their scrubs or write on a large poster in the break room to mark what they are letting go.

- It is human nature for staff to complain first, before they accept the new way of doing things. Avoid arguing with what you hear because it shuts down communication; rather, liberally use your active listening skills. Understanding is more important than agreement. Be transparent and let staff know if you don't know the answer; commit to finding out.

The significance of communication in the change and transition process should not be underestimated. It is essential in building broad support at both the organizational and local level. A key strategy is to be transparent and say everything more than once. Because of the amount of information that staff are exposed to, they need to hear it multiple times before they begin to pay attention. Bridges (2009) recommends a good rule of thumb as six times, six different ways, focused at the local level in very specific terms. For staff to see the outcome of the change and move through the transition, Bridges suggests four important communication guidelines:

1. Describe clearly where you are going with the change; if people understand what the *purpose* is, and the problem that led to the change, they will be better able to manage the uncertainty that comes with transition.

2. One outcome of communication is to leave staff with a clear, specific *picture* of what things will look like when the change is completed—What will the new workflow be? How will it look? What is it going to feel like? Who are the new players?

3. Explain the *plan* for change in as much detail as you have at the time; be transparent—if you don't know something, say so, and always follow with when, or what you will need, to answer their question at a future time.

4. People own what they create, so let staff know what you need from them, what *part* they will have, and where they will have choices or input.

Building Capacity

Building capacity refers to arming staff with the knowledge, skills, and resources to procure and judge the value of evidence and translate it into practice. Developing competency in using and applying EBP is best accomplished through education and direct practice gained through work in interprofessional teams.

Developing EBP Skills and Knowledge

The most popular format for EBP education programs at The Johns Hopkins Hospital is the one-day workshop. The morning session covers EBP concepts, the *JHNEBP Model and Guidelines*, and evidence searching and appraisal techniques. In the afternoon, attendees critique and appraise the evidence for an EBP question and decide, as a group, whether or not a practice change is warranted based on the evidence available to them. The one-day workshops have successfully been implemented in many settings outside of Johns Hopkins, including in rural, community, and nonteaching hospitals and other large academic medical centers. The educational topical outline for the one-day workshop is shown in Table 9.3.

Table 9.3   One-day Workshop Topics and Objectives

Subject Area	Objectives
Introduction to Evidence-Based Practice	Explain the origins of EBP Discuss importance of EBP Define EBP
Guidelines for Implementation	Describe JHNEBP Model Discuss plans for using the model Describe the steps in the process Discuss how to develop an answerable question
Appraising Evidence	Describe the different levels of evidence Determine where to look for evidence
Searching for Evidence	Discuss library services: How to have a search run by the library How to order articles Demonstrate how to do basic literature search
Appraising the Evidence Application	Provide explanation of the evidence appraisal forms Facilitate group appraisal/evaluation of assigned articles Discuss appraisal of level and quality of each article Complete Individual Evidence Summary Forms and synthesis and recommendation tools
Summarizing the Evidence and Beyond	Facilitate discussion of synthesis of the evidence Determine if practice changes are indicated based on the evidence Discuss fit, feasibility, and appropriateness of practice change Discuss how could the practice change can be implemented Discuss how changes can be evaluated

The Johns Hopkins Hospital nursing leadership also developed a competitive fellowship in EBP for staff nurses as an additional way to develop leaders and change champions for EBP. Two fellowships were budgeted yearly as a part-time opportunity for a nurse candidate, in partnership with a mentor, to develop EBP skills and complete a proposed project. The fellows use the *JHNEBP Model and Guidelines* to ask a practice question, critique and synthesize the literature, and translate their recommendations for practice improvement.

Interprofessional Collaboration

In today's team-focused health care environment, interprofessional collaboration for the evaluation and dissemination of evidence in the health care work setting is a high priority because many practice changes involve not only nurses, but also physicians, other allied health professionals, administrators, and policymakers. A conference held in February 2011 in Washington, DC, sponsored by the Health Resources and Services Administration (HRSA), Josiah Macy Jr. Foundation, Robert Wood Johnson Foundation, ABIM Foundation, and the Interprofessional Education Collaborative (IPEC), brought together more than 80 leaders from various health professions to review "Core Competencies for Interprofessional Collaborative Practice" (IPEC Expert Panel, 2011). The meeting's agenda focused on creating action strategies for the core competencies to transform health professional education and health care delivery in the United States. Competency Domain 4 supported the need for interprofessional teams to provide evidence-based care: "Apply relationship-building values and the principles of team dynamics to perform effectively in different team roles to plan and deliver patient-/population-centered care that is safe, timely, efficient, effective, and equitable" (p. 25). When EBP teams are being developed, interprofessional participation is key and the identification, and development of EBP mentors from the allied health professions should be considered.

The Johns Hopkins University School of Nursing

The Johns Hopkins University School of Nursing (JHUSON) recognized the need to prepare nurses with EBP knowledge and skills and adopted the *JHNEBP Model and Guidelines*, integrating both the model and PET process into didactic and clinical courses. In the baccalaureate research class, for example, real-life

EBP questions are generated from John Hopkins Hospital nursing units and given to the research instructor. As a course assignment, nursing students search and critique the available evidence from PubMed and CINAHL and prepare a summary of the literature for the unit to consider translating to practice. The master's program includes two courses in understanding and application of nursing research, Statistical Literacy and Reasoning in Nursing Research, and Application of Research to Practice. The first course focuses on enabling students to read and evaluate health care and nursing literature critically through understanding and use of statistics. The Application of Research to Practice course reviews the research process and helps students develop skills and knowledge needed to critique, rate, and synthesize the strength of available evidence and to discuss the translation of that evidence into practice.

EBP is also incorporated into master's-level clinical courses. To better see the application of the EBP process, nurse practitioner students identify a practice issue in their first clinical course and critique and synthesize the related literature throughout the three clinical courses. The PhD and Doctor of Nursing Practice (DNP) programs also incorporate evidence-based practice in their curricula. The PhD elective is Evidence-based Nursing. EBP is a foundational thread for the DNP program and two core courses emphasize that content. Additionally, DNP students complete systematic reviews of the literature in the focus area of their capstone projects. To more effectively integrate evidence-based practice concepts into the curriculum, several faculty development sessions have been held at the JHUSON. The faculty fast-tracked through the concepts and participated in an EBP project to experience using the model and the various tools.

Sustaining the Change

At the beginning of an EBP strategic initiative, the organization's leaders must support and sustain a change in how the organization approaches its work. The leaders, mentors, change champions, and those responsible for the initiative must continually listen to the staff and be responsive to their comments, questions, and complaints. For EBP to become fully adopted and integrated into the organization, the perception that changing practice will improve quality of care and make a difference in patients' lives must be felt by all staff. The passion will be palpable when EBP becomes a part of the daily routine. Therefore, sustaining the change requires an infrastructure that aligns staff expectations and organizational structures with the strategic vision and plan for a culture based on evidence.

Setting Expectations for EBP

Setting role expectations for EBP through development of job descriptions, orientation programs and materials, and performance evaluation tools is a first step in developing human capital for EBP and for hardwiring the culture of practice based on evidence. These personnel tools should be developed or revised to emphasize the staff's responsibility and accountability for making administrative and practice decisions to improve patient care outcomes and processes. The tools must be consistent across the employment continuum. For example, the job description should state what is expected of the nurse in terms of standards and measurement of competence; the orientation should introduce the nurse to the organization and how standards are upheld and competencies are developed at the organization; and the performance evaluation tool should measure the nurse's level of performance on the standards with specific measures of competence. Table 9.4 provides examples of standards of performance and competence from The Johns Hopkins Hospital department of nursing job descriptions.

Table 9.4   Excerpts from JHH Job Descriptions for Staff Nurses

CLINICAL PRACTICE

Nurse Clinician I: Applies a scientific basis or EBP approach to nursing practice.

1. Complies with changes in clinical practice and standards.

2. Participates in data collection when the opportunity is presented.

3. Poses relevant clinical questions when evidence and practice differ.

4. Consults appropriate experts when the basis for practice is questioned.

5. Uses appropriate resources to answer evidence-based practice questions.

Nurse Clinician II: Applies a scientific basis or EBP approach to nursing practice.

1. Seeks and/or articulates rationale and scientific basis for clinical practice or changes in standards.

2. Supports research-based clinical practice (teaches, role models, applies to own practices).

3. Participates in data collection when the opportunity is presented.

4. Identifies difference in practice and best evidence.

5. Generates clinical questions, searches evidence, and reviews evidence related to area of practice.

6. Consults appropriate experts to answer evidence-based practice questions.

7. Articulates evidence-based rationale for care.

Nurse Clinician III: Interprets research and uses scientific inquiry to validate and/or change clinical practice.

1. Evaluates research findings with potential implications for changing clinical practice, compares practice to findings, and takes appropriate action.

2. Designs tools and/or participates in data collection and other specific assignments (e.g., literature review) in the conduct of research when the opportunity presents.

3. Mentors staff to identify differences in practice and best evidence, generates clinical questions, searches evidence, reviews and critiques evidence related to area of clinical, administrative, or education practice.

4. Serves as a resource and mentor in evidence-based discussions articulating rationale for practice.

5. Participates in implementing evidence-based practice through role modeling and support of practice changes.

6. Incorporates EBP into daily patient care and leadership responsibilities.

7. Participates in/supports evidence-based practice projects within unit/department.

RESOURCES

Uses critical thinking and scientific inquiry to systematically and continually improve care and business processes and to achieve desired financial outcomes.

Committee Structure

The committee structure is designed to promote excellence in patient care, education, and research through

- Recruiting and retaining a diverse professional staff
- Establishing evidence-based standards of care and practice
- Promoting interprofessional quality improvement and research
- Advancing professional growth and development

The committees and their members took on the roles of EBP change champions and mentors for the department of nursing. Each committee serves a different but important role for implementing EBP throughout the organization, and annually, members develop an EBP question of importance to their committee work and goals for that year.

Table 9.5 describes EBP functions for the department of nursing professional practice committees.

Table 9.5   Department of Nursing Committee Functions Related to EBP

Committee	Functions
EBP Steering Committee	Establishes strategic initiatives for EBP within and external to The Johns Hopkins Hospital and The Johns Hopkins University School of Nursing
Clinical Quality Improvement Committee	Promotes evidence-based improvements in systems and processes of care to achieve safe, high-quality patient outcomes
Leadership Development Committee	Recommends and implements innovative evidence-based strategies for management and leadership practice
Research Committee	Supports discovery of new knowledge and translation into nursing practice

Committee	Functions
Standards of Care Committee	Promotes, develops, and maintains evidence-based standards of care
	Coaches departmental representatives in conducting their annual EBP project
	Recommends questions for JHUSON students to conduct EBP projects each semester
Standards of Practice Committee	Promotes, develops, and maintains evidence-based standards of professional practice

Communication Plan

A communication plan should be an integral part of both the EBP process and its sustainability. The plan should address the following:

- The goals of the communication
- Target audiences
- Available communication media
- Preferred frequency
- Important messages

Minimally, the goals for an EBP communication plan should focus on staff to increase awareness of the initiative, educate staff regarding their contribution, highlight and celebrate successes, and inform staff about EBP activities throughout the organization. Consider developing an EBP website within the organization's intranet. This website can be an excellent vehicle for communicating EBP information, including questions under consideration, projects in progress or completed, outcomes, and available EBP educational opportunities. The website can also serve as a snapshot and history of an organization's EBP activities and can be helpful when seeking or maintaining Magnet designation. Figure 9.3 shows The Johns Hopkins Hospital department of nursing EBP website.

Finally, the communication plan can use online surveys to involve staff by asking opinions about potential or completed work, maintaining a finger on the pulse of initiatives, and developing EBP messages. Messages can target the communication, link the initiative to the organization's mission, and give a consistent vision while providing new and varied information about the initiative.

After movement toward a supportive EBP environment begins, the biggest challenge is to keep the momentum going. To sustain the change, the staff must own the change and work to sustain it in a practice environment that values critical thinking and uses evidence for all administrative and clinical decision-making.

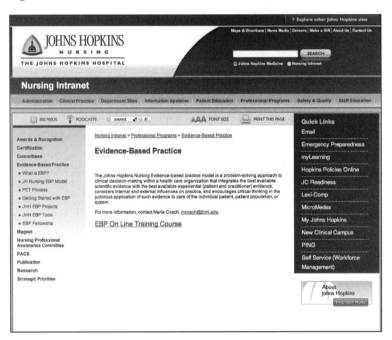

Figure 9.3   The Johns Hopkins Hospital department of nursing EBP website

As you allocate resources to an EBP initiative, some may raise questions about expenditures and the costs related to EBP. To sustain the work and value to the organization, you need to link EBP project work to organizational priorities. It is helpful to identify EBP projects that improve safety or risk management problems; address wide variations in practice or in clinical practice that is different from the community standard; or solve high-risk, high-volume, or high-cost problems. Consider asking the questions, "Is there evidence to support the organization's current practice? Are these the best achievable outcomes? Is there a way to be more efficient or cost-effective?" Improvements or benefits to the organization could result in any of these important areas if EPB work identified best practices to improve outcomes of care, decrease costs, or decrease risks associated with the problem. Another way of showing the cost-effectiveness of EBP work is to improve patient and/or staff satisfaction or health-related quality of life. Sustaining the change also involves developing an evaluation plan to identify process and outcome performance measures that monitor implementation, commitment, and results. The measures should determine the usefulness, satisfaction, and success of the EBP environment. Are the initiatives changing or supporting current practice? What best practices or exemplars have resulted? Has the organization saved money or become more efficient? What performance data show this is making a difference to the organization? The evaluation plan should include a timeline and triggers that would signal when a modification of the plan is necessary.

Summary

We have learned many lessons in the development, implementation, and continual refinement of the *JHNEBP Model and Guidelines*. The need to create a supportive EBP environment is one of the most important lessons. Essential to that effort is recognition of the importance of capacity building for EBP. A supportive leadership is essential to establish a culture of EBP, including the expansion of infrastructure and the allocation of resources such as time, money, and people to sustain the change. Leaders set priorities, facilitate the process, and set expectations. The development of local mentors and champions contributes to the successful implementation of EBP and helps overcome barriers and resistance to EBP.

A culture of critical thinking and ongoing learning creates an environment where evidence supports clinical and administrative decisions, assuring the highest quality of care by using evidence to promote optimal outcomes, reduce inappropriate variation in care, and promote patient and staff satisfaction. Working in an EBP environment changes the way nurses think about and approach that work. As the nursing staff develop expertise in the EBP process, their professional growth and engagement begins a personal and organizational trajectory leading to evidence-based decisions, a higher level of critical review of evidence, and engagement in the interprofessional team as valued contributors.

References

American Nurses Association (ANA). (2010). *Nursing: Scope and standards of nursing practice.* Washington, DC: American Nurses Publishing.

Balas, E., and Boren, S. A. (2000). Managing clinical knowledge for healthcare improvement. In J. Bemmel & A. T. McCray (Eds.), *Yearbook of Medical Informatics* (pp. 65-70). Bethesda, MD: National Library of Medicine.

Block, L. M., Claffey, C., Korow, M. K., & McCaffrey, R. (2005). The value of mentorship within nursing organizations. *Nursing Forum, 40*(4), 134-140.

Bridges, W. (2009). *Managing transitions: Making the most of change* (3rd ed.). Da Capo Press: PA.

Carroll, K. (2004). Mentoring: A human becoming perspective. *Nursing Science Quarterly, 17*(4), 318-322.

Dearholt, S. L., White, K. M., Newhouse, R., Pugh, L. C., & Poe, S. (2008). Educational strategies to develop evidence-based practice mentors. *Journal for Nurses in Staff Development*, 24(2), 53-59.

Estabrooks, C. (1998). Will evidence-based nursing practice make practice perfect? *Canadian Journal of Nursing Research*, 30(1), 15-36.

Greenhalgh, T., Robert, G., Macfarlane, F., Bate, P., & Kyriakidou, O. (2004). Diffusion of innovations in service organizations: Systematic review and recommendations. *The Milbank Quarterly, 82*(4), 581-629.

Institute of Medicine (IOM). (2001). *Crossing the quality chasm: A new health system for the 21st century*. Washington, DC: National Academy Press.

Institute of Medicine (IOM). (2003). *Health professions education: A bridge to quality.* Washington, DC: The National Academies Press.

Institute of Medicine (IOM). (2011). *The future of nursing: Leading change, advancing health.* Washington, DC: National Academy Press.

Interprofessional Education Collaborative (IPEC) Expert Panel. (2011). *Core competencies for interprofessional collaborative practice: Report of an expert panel.* Washington, D.C.: Interprofessional Education Collaborative.

McGlynn, E. A., Asch, S. M., Adams, J., Keesey, J., Hicks, J., DeCristofaro, A., & Kerr, E. A. (2003). The quality of health care delivered to adults in the United States. *New England Journal of Medicine, 348*(26), 2635-2645.

Newhouse, R., Dearholt, S., Poe, S., Pugh, L. C., & White. K. M. (2005). Evidence-based practice: A practical approach to implementation. *Journal of Nursing Administration, 35*(1), 35-40.

Newhouse, R. P. (2007). Creating infrastructure supportive of evidence-based nursing practice: Leadership strategies. *Worldviews on Evidence-Based Nursing, 4*(1), 21-29.

Owens, J. K., & Patton, J. G. (2003). Take a chance on nursing mentorships. *Nursing Education Perspectives, 24*(4), 198-204.

Pravikoff, D. S., Tanner, A. B., & Pierce, S. T. (2005). Readiness of U.S. nurses for evidence-based practice. *American Journal of Nursing, 105*(9), 40-5.

Schein, E. H. (2004). *Organizational culture and leadership* (3rd Ed.). San Francisco, CA: Jossey-Bass.

Titler, M. G., (2008). The evidence for evidence-based practice implementation. In R. G. Hughes (Ed.) *Patient Safety and Quality: An evidence-based handbook for nurses.* AHRQ Publication No. 08-0043, Rockville, MD: Agency for Healthcare Research and Quality.

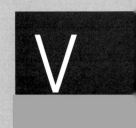

Exemplars

10

Exemplars

Maria Cvach, MS, RN, CCRN

The following section provides examples of how the Johns Hopkins Evidence-based Practice Model has been used in practice. These exemplars describe the work of nurses to answer clinical questions, determine need for practice change, or guide policy development using evidence.

1

Support Surfaces and Pressure Ulcers

Rachel N. Moseley, RN, CWON, CWCN
Cynthia A. Walker, RN, CWON
Mary Ann Greene, DNP, RN, NEA-BC
Zeina Khouri-Stevens, PhD, RN
Maria Koszalka, EdD, RN
Sarah J. M. Shaefer, PhD, RN

This exemplar describes the evolution of a practice issue identified when wound care nurses sought to decrease their patients' risk for pressure ulcers. It included a search for evidence and ultimately resulted in a cost analysis demonstrating the cost-effectiveness of replacing all mattresses on the adult medical/surgical units. This exemplar describes the evidence-based practice (EBP) process while not recommending a specific product.

Practice Question

Hospital protocol requires that adult medical/surgical patients at risk for pressure ulcer development (Braden Scale score of 18 or less) be placed on the appropriate support surface to prevent pressure ulcers. Patients with a Braden score of 16 or less were placed on a low air loss (or similar) mattress; patients with Braden scores of 17 or 18 were placed on a specific mattress. Both products were either single mattress overlays or rented mattresses. Patients were on standard mattresses until these more appropriate mattresses were available.

Pressure ulcers can develop within six to 12 hours in healthy individuals and in less than two hours in a debilitated patient. Data from 31 medical/surgical patients revealed the average time between patient risk assessment and mattress delivery was 48 hours. Time was calculated based on entry of Braden Scale into the electronic medical record, online order for appropriate mattress, and mattress application to the bed frame. This time lag, primarily due to the labor-intensive process of changing a mattress while trying to maintain patient comfort, increased the patient's risk for developing a pressure ulcer. The Wound, Ostomy, and Continence Nurses Society (WOCN), in *Guideline for Prevention and*

Management of Pressure Ulcers, along with the National Pressure Ulcer Advisory Panel (NPUAP) in "Pressure Ulcer Prevention Points," state that at-risk individuals should be placed on a pressure redistribution surface rather than a generic hospital mattress. Pressure ulcers are preventable and, after they develop, are expensive to treat. The Centers for Medicare and Medicaid Services consider stage III and IV hospital-acquired pressure ulcers as a *"never event"* medical error. *Never events* are not reimbursable at the higher rate associated with their care. Though support surfaces are only one aspect of pressure ulcer prevention, providing an advanced pressure redistribution surface the moment the patient arrives on the floor demonstrates a proactive, not reactive, approach to preventing pressure ulcers.

The practice problem was that the mattress and overlay system contributed to a delay in immediate availability of an appropriate pressure redistribution surface. The wound care nurses sought to find a way to minimize or eliminate the delay in surface availability.

The practice question was, "Can the purchase of an advanced therapeutic support surface as the standard mattress for medical/surgical unit beds provide effective and timely pressure redistribution surfaces and be cost effective for the facility compared to the current practice of using mattresses and overlays?"

Evidence

The evidence search included literature, professional organization standards of practice, a survey of Magnet hospital wound care nurses, and a financial analysis. A Cochrane review of 53 studies, both randomized controlled trials (RCTs) and quasi-experimental, found that pressure ulcers were reduced in people at risk (RR 0.40; 95% CI 0.21 to 0.74) when alternatives to standard hospital foam mattresses were used. Though specific product results are mixed, the review recommended that patients with a high risk of developing pressure ulcers use higher specification foam mattresses rather than standard hospital mattresses.

A review of the recommendations from the NPUAP, WOCN, and The Advisory Board Company show use of pressure redistribution surfaces should be part of a hospital's protocol. However, of the more than 200 types of surfaces available, no one surface is shown to be superior to another.

To validate current practice and experience with support surfaces, 70 wound care registered nurse specialists from east coast Magnet hospitals were surveyed with a 29% response rate. These nurses were asked about type of support surface used, ownership or rental status, pressure ulcer rate changes, and opinion of importance of support surface to prevent ulcers. Importance of the support surface was rated 4.53 to 5.00 on a 5-point Likert scale (5 = most important) for the prevention of pressure ulcers. The majority of respondents owned and/or rented support surfaces and reported satisfaction with the specific products used and a decrease in pressure ulcers.

Though the need for changes in mattresses for effective support system was indicated, evidence on specific product recommendations was limited. Manufacturer's claims regarding specific products should be independently validated. A case study provided in The Advisory Board Company Nursing Executive Center, "Safeguarding Against Nursing Never Events," showed a reduction in the prevalence of pressure ulcers from 10.4% to 4.3% with the system-wide deployment of an advanced support surface at Intermountain Healthcare in Utah. The case study also reported an estimated cost savings of $23.5 million over one year for a 21-hospital system. Clearly, using an advanced therapeutic support surface as soon as possible is ideal; however, choosing the appropriate surface may be more difficult because the evidence varies as to which surface is superior.

The hospital conducted a product evaluation to determine if the advanced support surface mattresses were easy to work with and comfortable for the patient. This evaluation was not designed to determine if pressure ulcer prevalence would decrease. No major issues were noted with the product evaluation. Other hospitals in the health system currently using the advanced mattresses have not reported any major issues.

The annual cost for rental, single use overlays, and routine mattress replacement for the adult medical/surgical units was $122,839. The purchase of 196 advanced therapeutic support mattresses for adult medical/surgical beds was approximately $136,559. Savings were $200 monthly, after the initial purchase of mattresses and deductions for rental costs, with a projected 5-year savings of $391,111.

Translation

The evidence indicated that patients at high risk for pressure ulcers require a pressure redistribution support surface at admission. There appeared to be an excessive delay in providing this to patients when rental was required. One cost-effective solution was to replace all mattresses with the pressure redistribution support surface. Based on evidence from this project, the Vice President for Patient Care Services funded new mattresses. With this implementation, the hospital had a seen an 8% reduction in hospital-acquired pressure ulcer (HAPU) prevalence rates over six reporting quarters for the National Database of Nursing Quality Indicators (NDNQI). The second quarter reflected these efforts with no unit-acquired pressure ulcers in any of the NDNQI reportable units. The second quarter also marked a record low HAPU prevalence of 2.08%. Wound team members have been energized by these results and continue aggressive efforts to maintain safety and preserve skin for our patients.

Summary

Pressure ulcers have long been associated with the quality of nursing care and preventing them has been a persistent and pervasive nursing concern. Florence Nightingale wrote in 1859, "If he has a bedsore, it's generally not the fault of the disease, but of the nursing." With the introduction of a pressure redistribution support surface, patients can be protected from hospital-acquired pressure ulcers.

2

Use of Evidence-Based Practice Model by a Professional Nursing Association

Paula Graling, DrNP, CNS, RN, CNOR

The Association of periOperative Registered Nurses (AORN) is a professional nursing association established in 1954. Its mission is to promote safety and optimal outcomes for patients undergoing operative and other invasive procedures by providing practice support and professional development opportunities to perioperative nurses. Currently, AORN serves over 40,000 members across the globe.

AORN Recommended Practices represent the Association's official position on what is believed to be an optimal level of patient care within surgical and invasive procedure settings. The recommendations are broad statements intended to guide policy and procedure development in specific work environments and are intended to describe best perioperative nursing practices to promote patient and healthcare worker safety. These documents are based on principles of nursing science, microbiology, research, review of scientific literature, and the opinions of knowledgeable experts.

Practice Issue

The use of scientific evidence to support national recommendations about clinical decisions has become an expectation of multidisciplinary health care organizations. Evidence-based practice (EBP) is an essential method of improving patient care by promoting decisions based on scientific evidence rather than on the opinion of the individual health care provider. AORN members reported difficulty engaging in discussions with practitioners in other disciplines about the evidence behind the recommended practices. Though a robust list of references has always been provided with each recommended practice, individual references have never been assessed for their quality and strength. The AORN Board of Directors formed a task force, led by Dr. Victoria Steelman, to evaluate a methodology that would direct the review of evidence used in creating a recommended practice and select a method to rate the overall strength of the evidence. Many evidence-rating methods were available, but the best method for communicating the strength of scientific evidence supporting AORN recommendations had not been identified prior to the work of the task force in 2010.

Evidence

The task force completed its work in June of 2010 and recommended a methodology for incorporating evidence rating into AORN documents. The redesign of the Recommended Practices process utilizes a systems approach.

- Each Recommended Practice under review focuses on a specific question or topic.

- A comprehensive search strategy is conducted by a research librarian employed by the Association.

- As relevant studies are located, they are critically appraised using the Johns Hopkins Nursing Evidence-based Practice (JHNEBP) Model. The appraisal team consists of a perioperative nursing practice specialist in charge of authoring the document, an identified subject matter expert who is often the second author, a nurse researcher, and a member of the Recommended Practice Advisory Board. AORN is fortunate to have an advisory board consisting not only of expert perioperative nurses, but also physicians and other colleagues representing members of the surgical team.

- After the studies are appraised using either the research or non-research appraisal tools, the collective evidence is synthesized into a summary table and rated using the Oncology Nursing Society *Putting Evidence into Practice (PEP)* schema. Factors considered in review of collective evidence are the quality of research, quantity of similar studies on a given topic, and consistency of results supporting a recommendation.

The transparency of the process allows AORN to demonstrate the strength of the evidence supporting the Recommended Practice and promote adoption of the recommendation in clinical practice.

Translation

Since mid-2011, all new Recommended Practices under review or development begin with an extensive literature search. The project leader submits a search request to the AORN research librarian. The strategy used to conduct the literature search is documented for retrievability. Articles identified by the search are provided to the project team for evaluation. The appraisal team consists of at least four individuals: a nurse specialist from AORN, a subject matter expert, a nurse researcher, and an advisory board member. All relevant literature is independently evaluated and appraised according to the strength and quality of the evidence using the JHNEBP Model Evidence Appraisal tools. Each individual enters their scores into an electronic database. Conference calls are utilized to discuss the appraisal scores given by each team member and to establish consensus of appraisal rankings. The collective evidence supporting each intervention within a specific Recommended Practice is then summarized and used to rate the strength of the evidence using the PEP schema. The PEP schema includes six levels for rating the *collective* evidence supporting a recommendation:

- Recommended for practice
- Likely to be effective
- Benefits balanced with harm
- Effectiveness not established
- Effectiveness unlikely
- Not recommended for practice

As the literature search is being conducted, the primary author constructs an initial draft of the Recommended Practice based on current trends in practice. The results of the literature search may validate current trends for inclusion in the subsequent drafts or may identify gaps in knowledge that were not previously identified. The literature search may also identify current practice trends that are no longer supported by the evidence.

Summary

The ability to incorporate evidence-based nursing into clinical care requires a basic understanding of the main research designs underlying the published evidence. The applicability of the JHNEBP Model for appraisal of evidence linked to AORN Recommended Practices is based on its methodology allowing consideration of all types of evidence for review. Multiple randomized clinical trials are not often available to guide clinical practice decisions. Use of lower levels of evidence to guide decision-making may be needed when true randomized control trials are unavailable. Perioperative nurses have a professional responsibility to use EBP; appraisal of studies and rating of evidence provide valuable information to readers and help with clinical discussions and decision-making.

The successful implementation of an evidence-based practice model for AORN will depend on the ability to appraise individual pieces of evidence and collectively rate the strength of the evidence regarding specific interventions by the surgical team. Confidence in using this process and the related tools will come only with diligent practice and application over the next few years. The opportunity provided by using this process will allow AORN to identify gaps in the literature that direct future perioperative research efforts.

3

Placing Patients Taking Oral Antiplatelet Medications on Bleeding Precautions

Maria Cvach, MS, RN, CCRN
Emily Munchel, RN, CPN

This exemplar, conducted by a Standards of Care Committee, demonstrates how a committee investigated whether adult patients should be placed on bleeding precautions to minimize risk for bleeding injury. This project resulted in a policy amendment that places patients taking multiple antiplatelet medications on bleeding precautions.

Practice Question

Patients who are at risk of bleeding and sustain a fall can experience serious injury. For this reason, the Fall Advisory Task Force at the hospital recently added a fall injury assessment requirement for adult inpatients. Bleeding risk is one of the fall injury assessment parameters. Patients who are considered to be at risk of bleeding include those taking anticoagulant and thrombolytic medication, as well as patients with various conditions such as thrombocytopenia and hemophilia. The practice concern was that the current bleeding precautions protocol did not include patients receiving oral antiplatelet drugs, except under specific circumstances (e.g., aspirin for intracranial surgery patients).

The Nursing Standards of Care (SOC) Committee decided to review the evidence regarding oral antiplatelet drugs and risk of bleeding as their annual EBP project. The outcome was to determine if adult inpatients taking oral antiplatelet medication should be placed on bleeding precautions to minimize risk for bleeding injury.

The EBP team consisted of a nursing EBP fellow, nurse leaders, and department nursing representatives such as bedside nurses, nurse managers, and nurse educators. The practice question was, "Will placing adult inpatients receiving aspirin or other oral anti-platelet agents on bleeding precautions decrease bleeding injury?"

Evidence

The nursing EBP fellow and a medical librarian conducted separate searches of various databases including PubMed, Cumulative Index to Nursing and Allied Health Literature (CINAHL), Scopus, and Embase. The search terms used were

- *Antiplatelet* AND *fall injury*

- *Antiplatelet* AND *bleeding precautions*

- *Aspirin* AND *fall injury*

- *Bleeding precautions* AND *fall risk*

- *Aspirin* AND *bleeding precautions*

The initial search yielded over 50 articles. These were narrowed down by the EBP team project leader to 12 relevant articles. The 20 SOC members were divided into four groups and each group was assigned a set of three articles to read; each member within a group read the same articles. The small groups, led by an EBP mentor, discussed, appraised, and presented findings to the entire group. Eleven of the articles appraised were applicable to the EBP question.

Using tools from the JHNEBP Model, the SOC committee found the evidence to be consistent, with good-to-high quality and strength. Findings indicated that patients who are on two or more oral antiplatelet drugs are at a greater risk for bleeding than those who are prescribed only one antiplatelet agent. Aspirin was found to increase GI bleeding risk at both low (70–100 mg) and high (> 100 mg) doses, but was not found to cause major injury on its own.

Translation

The SOC Committee discussed the implications of placing additional patients on bleeding precautions. Committee members and pharmacy staff expressed concern that placing too many patients on bleeding precautions may result in staff minimizing or ignoring the importance of this precaution. The SOC Committee considered the evidence, along with the staff and pharmacy preferences, in determining the implementation path. The team did not find a compelling reason to add "patients taking a single oral dose of antiplatelet medication" to the list of indicators for use of the bleeding precautions protocol. However, the team did agree that the protocol should be amended to include patients who were taking two or more oral antiplatelet drugs as an indicator for bleeding precautions. In addition, the team agreed that patients with a history of GI bleed who are prescribed aspirin also should be placed on bleeding precautions. These recommendations were used to reverse the policy.

Summary

The findings from this EBP process were disseminated to the nursing staff through education about the protocol changes. Self-audits are conducted periodically to determine compliance with implementing bleeding precautions. Outcomes are measured through the hospital's incident reporting process.

Fall Injury Risk Assessment

Maria Cvach, MS, RN, CCRN
Patricia B. Dawson, MSN, RN

Although much research on fall risk assessment and fall prevention in acute care inpatient settings exists, relatively little research specifically addresses factors that predispose the patient to injury from falls. After completing an EBP project, a Fall Prevention Subcommittee conducted a pilot study to determine the effectiveness of an injury risk factor assessment in decreasing serious injury from falls before incorporating this assessment into the fall prevention protocol.

Practice Question

This problem surfaced as a practice concern because costs associated with injury from falls while hospitalized are substantial. In addition, fall injury is associated with reduced mobility and independence and with increased mortality in the elderly. Though most hospitals use assessment tools to predict fall risk, few hospitals assess risk of injury from a fall and target interventions based on a fall injury risk assessment. For this reason, the Fall Prevention Subcommittee decided to review evidence related to fall injury assessment. The practice question posed was, "Will the assessment of fall injury risk factors and implementation of appropriate interventions decrease serious injury from falls in the adult acute care setting?"

Evidence

A literature search was conducted by several members of the Fall Prevention Subcommittee and a nursing EBP fellow. The following databases were searched: CINAHL, PubMed, the Cochrane Database of Systematic Reviews, Google Scholar, and the National Guideline Clearinghouse. The search terms used included *fall injury risk, anticoagulation therapies, activities of daily living, aged, depressive disorder, cognitive disorder, postoperative complications, subdural hematoma, pain,* and *postoperative diagnosis.*

This EBP project was used as the practice problem in the semi-annual EBP workshop; article appraisals were completed by participants under the leadership of EBP mentors. Sixteen nurse participants were divided into four groups for article review; each group member read the same set of three articles. Of the 12 articles critiqued and appraised, seven were applicable to the EBP practice question, including two experimental studies, four non-experimental studies, and one clinical practice guideline. The evidence identified the following fall injury risk factors:

- Elderly (advanced age)

- Female gender

- Bleeding risk, particularly from antiplatelet medication

- Cognitive impairment or mini-mental score of less than 26

- Body mass index (BMI) less than 22

- Decreased bone density and vitamin D deficiency

- Two or more chronic medical diseases

These findings were submitted to the Fall Prevention Subcommittee for review and consideration in developing a fall injury risk assessment. After review, the committee decided several of the factors identified could be grouped together. For example, BMI less than 22, decreased bone density, and vitamin D deficiency were all related to a patient's fracture risk. Therefore, one of the criteria selected for incorporation into a fall injury risk assessment was fracture risk. Another category recommended for inclusion was bleeding risk. Though advanced age was identified in several articles as a fall injury risk factor, the definition of advanced age was inconsistently reported. After reviewing the literature, the committee agreed that age greater than 80 should be used as the final parameter. The group did not feel that two risk factors had clinical significance: female gender and two or more chronic diseases. The committee's rationale for not including these was that the number of people in these categories was too great and would cause over prediction of risk.

Translation

Having selected the fall injury assessment parameters of age greater than 80, bleeding risk, and fracture risk, the Fall Prevention Subcommittee decided to pilot assessment of these parameters over a 6-week period on two hospital units to test the feasibility of incorporating them into the fall risk assessment and intervention process. These two units, a cardiac surgical step-down and a transplant surgical unit, were selected because their unit fall and fall injury rates were sporadically higher than those of other hospital units. In addition, these units used an electronic clinical documentation system that allowed for programming the assessment and interventions into the electronic medical record. In the pilot, nurses completed the assessment of fall injury risk in conjunction with their routine fall risk assessment using The Johns Hopkins Fall Risk Assessment Tool. The existing fall prevention protocol had three categories of risk interventions based on low, moderate, or high fall risk. The pilot protocol added another three categories of risk interventions: (a) low fall with positive injury risk, (b) moderate fall with positive injury risk, and (c) high fall with positive injury risk. In both the existing and pilot protocols, the most time- and cost-intensive preventive interventions were prioritized to patients at greatest fall and fall injury risk. For example, the use of patient safety attendants was recommended for patients in the high risk to falls and positive injury risk categories. A nurse champion from each unit participated in the pilot planning, and development and delivery of education to the other nurses on the unit.

Effectiveness of fall injury interventions was closely tied to nurses' perception of usability and value to improving patient safety. To that end, the pilot evaluated compliance with documentation of the fall injury risk assessment and interventions, staff feedback on how easy the process was to complete, and how valuable staff found the information in planning care.

Review of data from the 6-week pilot revealed fall assessment and fall injury risk were both completed in 79% of the assessments. Staff used the combination of the fall risk and fall injury risk factors, when completed together, to assign the appropriate risk category for 86% of those assessments. Staff surveys revealed 82% of respondents completed injury risk assessments in two minutes or less. Fifty-four percent agreed that assessing and highlighting fall injury risk factors added value to their care planning. Focus groups found that many staff (particularly on the cardiac unit with a majority of patients on antiplatelets) wanted more specificity on the bleeding risk criteria. Nurses from both units noted the six categories of fall interventions, computer screen design, and multiple layers of interventions made documentation too cumbersome. Pilot unit fall event data revealed one unit had no falls during the 6 weeks before or during the pilot, and the other unit had a decrease in the fall and fall injury events between pre-pilot and pilot periods.

Summary

The Fall Prevention Subcommittee voted to proceed with house-wide integration of fall injury risk assessment into the fall prevention protocol. The pilot provided justification for additional programming to reconfigure fall assessment and protocol documentation in the electronic medical record. Ongoing monitoring for serious injuries due to falls is incorporated in the hospital's quality improvement program.

Preventing Pediatric Infiltrates

Lori D. Van Gosen, MSN, RN, CRNI

This exemplar describes an EBP project conducted by pediatric nurses to determine the best practices of preventing infiltrates in the pediatric population. The nurses identified three factors associated with infiltrate prevention: assessment, securement, and placement. The team developed an educational plan to disseminate their findings and next steps were identified.

Practice Question

Pediatric intravenous (IV) infiltrates are an ongoing practice concern and are related, in part, to catheter size, fluid composition, site selection, and a child's developmental level. Consequences of IV infiltrates can be as simple as slight swelling or severe enough to require surgery. IV management varied across units in the Children's Center, and best practice strategies needed to be identified.

An EBP team was assembled, led by an EBP fellow who is also the senior nurse for the Pediatric Vascular Access Team. Other team members included staff nurses from the infant unit, school-age unit, and NICU. The practice question was, "What are the best practices to prevent IV infiltrates in the pediatric population?"

Evidence

A literature search was conducted using PubMed, CINAHL, Cochrane, www.guidelines.gov, and Google Scholar. In the pediatric literature, 18 articles were appraised; two random controlled trials and eight expert opinions were relevant to the EBP question. In the adult literature, 28 articles were appraised with three identified as adding relevant information. All of the adult articles were identified as expert opinion. After the literature appraisal, the best practice

recommendations identified were *assessment, securement,* and *placement.*
Assessment practices included:

- Assessing the IV site every hour for swelling, redness, leaking, and blanching

- Not relying solely on the infusion pump as an indication of building pressure

- Verifying that medication and fluid is appropriate for the line location

- Identifying when more thoroughly diluting caustic IV push medications can help save the vein sensitivity

- Recognizing the most opportune time for good assessment is at change of shift and when occupancy rates rise above average because both of these times have shown an increase in rates of infiltration

- Recognizing extra guidance and support is needed for new staff to identify infiltrations early and prevent infiltrate injuries

Securement recommendations included

- Ensuring the insertion site is fixed firmly to reduce catheter movement in the vein

- Applying the tape so it is secure yet not so tight that it obstructs venous flow

- Making certain that the insertion site is always visible

Placement recommendations included

- Reducing endothelial damage by using appropriate catheter size, e.g., not placing a large IV in a small vein

- Avoiding areas of flexion when possible; if necessary, applying an arm or foot board

- Avoid placing a new IV in a site near a previous infiltration

Translation

The EBP team, concerned about staff buy-in, incorporated the Quality Improvement Committee as part of the team. This provided representation from every unit in the Children's Center. The EBP process was repeated with the reformed group and best practice recommendations discussed. A nurse educator also joined the team to assist with strategies for communicating the practice changes to staff.

Educational Plans

- A Palpating, Inspecting, Validating (P.I.V.) educational sheet was created to summarize the hourly assessment procedure of the IV site.

- In conjunction with pharmacy, a color-coded educational sheet was created to identify which medications were more damaging to vessels and thus needed to be more diligently monitored.

- The acronym SISI—standing for Stage, Infusate, Securement, Intervention—was created and posted on workstation computers to guide nurses on procedures to consistently report infiltrates.

- PowerPoint slides were created to educate nurses on how to stage infiltrates to ensure consistency throughout the Children's Center.

- The Standards of Care Committee was consulted to ensure that the peripheral IV protocol was revised to reflect the EBP recommendations.

Summary

The outcome measure of the number of infiltrates was difficult to obtain. Staff did not consistently report infiltrates. The most accurate information regarding the number of infiltrates was collected by the Pediatric Vascular Access Team when an IV restart was performed; the team tracked how many restarts were due to an infiltrate. Although this method may not capture all of the instances, it is useful in evaluating the effectiveness of the recommendations. As a next step, the EBP team plans a trial involving securement devices to see which is the most effective at reducing infiltrate rates and is easiest to use.

6

The Frequency of Manufactured Intravenous Fluid Bag Replacement

Emily Munchel, RN, CPN
Regina Hendrix, MSN, MPA, RN-BC,
Keisha Perrin, RN
Shilta Subhas, MS, RN
Kathleen Wagner-Kosmakos, MS, RN

This exemplar describes an EBP project conducted by an interprofessional team to address variation in practice between adult and pediatric units for IV fluid bag replacement. The project outcomes resulted in a practice change that would save the hospital money on tubing supplies, save nursing time and decrease the risk of infection through decreased IV line manipulation.

Practice Question

Protocols and practices for manufactured intravenous (IV) fluid bag replacement varied among the patient care units depending on patient age or route of administration. Manufactured IV fluid bags are those used exactly as they are received from the manufacturer, without additives by in-house pharmacists or nurses. This can include NSS, D5 ½ NSS, LR, or KCL. Current practice, according to the hospital's Adult Venous Access Device (VAD) protocol was to leave IV tubing in place for 96 hours and change manufactured IV fluid every 24 hours; arterial line manufactured IV bags were changed every 96 hours. The Pediatric VAD protocol directed nurses to change the IV tubing and manufactured IV fluid together every 72 hours or sooner if the fluid administration was completed. Given the nursing time and costs involved in IV maintenance, clinicians recognized the need for standardization throughout the institution. An interprofessional team was assembled to conduct an evidence-based practice (EBP) project to address the problem of lack of consistency between adult and pediatric units for IV fluid bag replacement. Team members included nurses from pediatrics, adult medicine, oncology and hematology, with consultation from an infection control specialist from Hospital

Epidemiology and Infection Control (HEIC). The background practice question posed was: "What is the best practice for how often a manufactured IV fluid bag should be changed?"

Evidence

A literature search was conducted by using the Cumulative Index to Nursing and Allied Health Literature (CINAHL), PubMed, and Embase with the assistance of a medical librarian. Forty-two articles were identified through the search. Of the 16 articles appraised, the group determined that 11 were applicable to the EBP question. Two team members appraised each article using the tools from the Johns Hopkins Nursing Evidence-Based Practice (JHNEBP) Model. Two questions were posed to a proprietary hospital consortium Listserv where academic medical centers query peer institutions. The questions were: "What is your hospital protocol for the frequency of changing manufacturer-supplied IV fluid bags such as Normal Saline and D5W?" and "What is your hospital protocol for the frequency of changing heparinized and non-heparinized flush bags?" The information received was recorded on the Individual Evidence Summary Tool as experiential evidence (Level V). The majority of institutions that responded to this query had protocols for changing manufacturer-supplied IV fluid bags and flush bags similar to the hospital's policy. The EBP team completed the Synthesis and Recommendations Tool, which included five experimental studies, one quasi-experimental study, and four non-experimental or qualitative studies. Additionally, there were three clinical practice guidelines published by the Centers for Disease Control (CDC) and three articles based on expert opinion, two of which were the adult and pediatric venous access device protocols used at the hospital. All of the evidence appraised was given a high or good quality rating.

The evidence review showed three consistent themes. First, the more manipulation that occurs with an IV line, the greater the risk of contamination; repeated entry to an IV line is a potential means of introducing bacteria into that administration set. Second, IV systems should not be violated from the initial set-up until the treatment is discontinued, if possible. And third, the optimal interval for routine IV set replacement is 72 hours and 96 hours for replacement of disposable arterial transducer sets.

Translation

Based on the evidence found, the recommendation was made that IV tubing and manufactured IV bags would be changed together, every 72 hours. This practice change would save the hospital money on wasted tubing supplies. It would also save nursing time and decrease the risk of infection through decreased IV line manipulation. The next step was to present a summary of the findings and recommendations to HEIC and the Venous Access Device (VAD) committees for review. Concurrent to the dissemination of the EBP findings, the 2011 CDC Guidelines were published. The VAD committee and HEIC combined the team's EBP evidence with these new guidelines, and determined that IV tubing and manufactured IV bags could be changed together every 96 hours. This change was incorporated into the hospital's updated Adult VAD protocol.

Summary

This project has had a positive impact on a large number of nurses and patients at the hospital. Previously, it could take a nurse as long as an hour a day to change all of her patients' IV fluid bags. Now that hour can be devoted to other aspects of patient care. As a team, nurses were able to use the JHNEBP model to guide decision-making within the institution. The success of this project taught the team that the EBP process is an effective way to make change within the organization and fostered a positive attitude towards EBP among hospital staff.

Ankyloglossia, Frenotomy, and Breast Feeding

Deborah Dixon, RN, IBCLC
Kathleen White, PhD, RN, NEA-BC, FAAN

This exemplar discusses a practice concern raised by the nursing staff. It describes key lessons learned when dealing with an interprofessional team, especially with a practice question of concern to our physician colleagues. It concludes with a discussion of the translation possibilities when a search reveals limited strong scientific evidence.

Practice Question

The lactation specialist team at a nonteaching, community hospital encountered infants assessed to have a congenital anomaly called ankyloglossia or "tongue-tie." This occurred in about 4.6% of the newborn infant population at their facility. These newborns are usually unable to breastfeed properly. Some are completely unable to attach to the mother's nipple; others are able to attach, but less efficiently than babies with unrestricted tongue motion, and are unable to transfer enough milk to be satisfied. Additionally, ankyloglossia can cause severe nipple trauma to the mother. The treatment most useful in newborns is called frenotomy, a snipping of the tongue-tie. The lactation team's experience had shown that if frenotomy was performed within the first 72 hours of life, the newborn was able to latch on properly, transfer the mother's milk, and minimize nipple discomfort. About 60% of the pediatricians at the facility routinely ordered frenotomy performed when ankyloglossia was assessed by the lactation nurses. However, 40% of the pediatricians did not, so this fact suggested a review of the evidence for dealing with ankyloglossia.

One private pediatrician agreed to join the team to represent the views of the 60% of pediatricians generally in favor of treating ankyloglossia with frenotomy. The lactation team and nursery nurses viewed this as a positive sign and tried to schedule a team meeting to discuss the practice question. They found, however, that the physician could not meet with them for almost three months. The lesson learned from this experience was not to be discouraged with delay like this; forming an interprofessional team is often a challenge. It is suggested, when confirming the first meeting, to also schedule additional meetings at two–three-week intervals to keep the project moving. In the meantime, the lactation team, anxious to get the work underway, proceeded to define the practice question, "What are the best practices to treat ankyloglossia?"

Evidence

The lactation specialist team leader and two faculty members from the Johns Hopkins University School of Nursing who had faculty practices at the hospital conducted an evidence review in CINAHL and PubMed based on the practice question. The terms used for the search were *ankyloglossia*, *treatment*, and *frenotomy*. This search yielded 40 articles. These articles were acquired and assembled for discussion and critique. At the first team meeting, however, the pediatrician disagreed with the practice question. He suggested the other pediatricians would be more interested in the question, "What are risks and benefits of frenotomy in newborn with ankyloglossia?" Another valuable lesson in teamwork learned was to involve the interprofessional team from the very beginning in defining the problem and scope of the project. This ensures agreement on the practice question among all members of the team.

A second search of evidence for the new practice question used the terms *ankyloglossia, frenotomy, risks, benefits*, and *complications*. This search yielded 27 pieces of evidence from CINAHL and PubMed that the team reviewed to inform the practice question:

- Four level I (experimental studies)
- Two level II (quasi-experimental studies)
- Five level III (non-experimental studies)
- Five level IV (articles written by nationally recognized experts based on scientific evidence)
- Eleven level V (articles written by experts based on their experience)

The level I studies, all of good quality, confirmed that ankyloglossia adversely affects breastfeeding, and those identified as tongue-tied were three times as likely as a control group to be bottle fed at one week. It was also interesting that the studies reported a 4.8–5% incidence of ankyloglossia, similar to the incidence rate at the facility.

The level II evidence, also rated at good quality, reported a 96% inter-rater reliability for use of the Hazelbaker Assessment Tool to measure lingual frenulum function.

The level III evidence confirmed the usefulness of the Hazelbaker Assessment Tool to measure ankyloglossia. This level of evidence also reported on the poor latch and nipple pain associated with ankyloglossia. In addition, level III evidence reported frenotomy being performed with two studies reporting no complications after the procedure and improvement in the newborn's ability to latch on to the breast; frenotomy was recommended as treatment for ankyloglossia to improve the newborn's ability to breastfeed.

Level IV evidence reported on frenotomy as a simple, safe, and low-risk procedure. Level V evidence described a laser procedure for tight frenulum, reported speech problems if frenulum remains tight, and discussed dental problems and social issues related to speech problems if the tongue-tie persists. Several case reports at this level reported frenotomy as safe and effective with no complications, with only one case in 44 reporting bleeding and pain.

The synthesis of the evidence review included

- Ankyloglossia adversely affects breastfeeding, causes nipple pain and poor latch
- Infants identified as tongue-tied were three times as likely as the control group to be bottle fed at one week
- Some evidence suggests that ankyloglossia causes speech and social issues later in childhood
- The Hazelbaker Assessment Tool for lingual frenulum function had a 96% inter-rater reliability for assessment

- Frenotomy was reported as safe and effective with no complications in many case reports
- Limited controlled scientific evidence for frenotomy exists

Translation

Translation of this evidence review has been two-pronged. First, the evidence summary was presented at the pediatrician department staff meeting. Again, it took over three months to schedule the summary presentation. The team had to be reminded not to get discouraged with the delay; dissemination of evidence review is extremely important and influential in changing practice or behavior. The results of the project, with limited strong scientific evidence promoting frenotomy, were shared with the pediatricians. The lactation team hoped to raise awareness so open discussion of treatment options could occur when a newborn was assessed to have ankyloglossia.

Second, at the conclusion of this project, the lactation team leader took a new position as a Lactation Consultant Coordinator within an affiliate hospital. In this position, she has presented the evidence review to pediatric nurse practitioners, neonatologists, obstetric and pediatric residents, and other lactation specialists. She has improved the team's awareness of ankyloglossia and frenotomy as a treatment. A lactation training seminar has taught the nurses, residents, and nurse practitioners to assess infant's latch, suck, and anatomy of tongue so that if ankyloglossia is found on assessment, the oral surgeon can be notified for a consult. In addition, if frenotomy is performed, before and after weights are assessed for the newborn, and the mother's nipple pain is also assessed. Finally, because the evidence was not strong enough for a clear practice change, a research study was initiated to assess the effects of early ankyloglossia detection, early frenotomy treatment, and how these affect infants' growth and mothers' breastfeeding comfort.

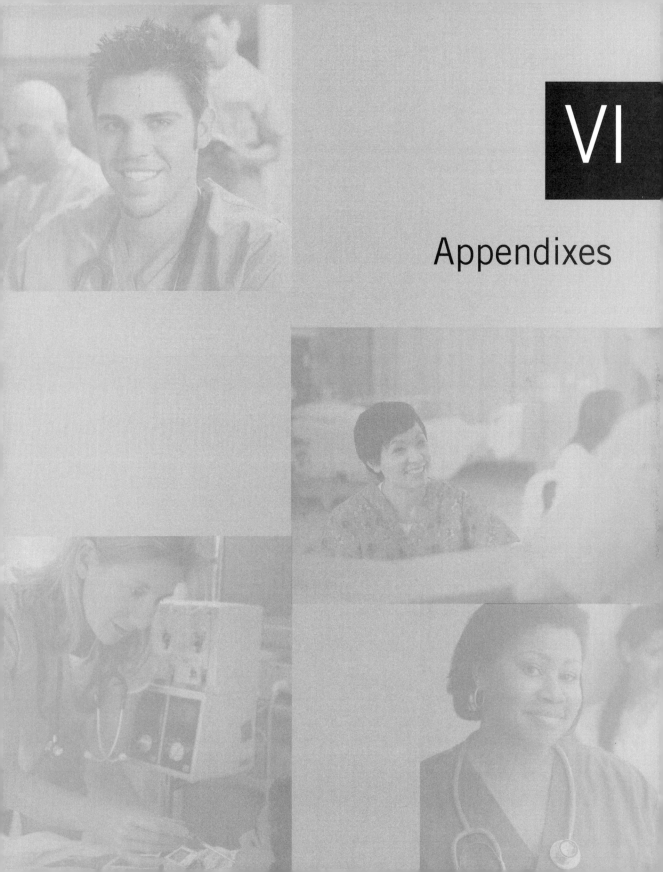

VI

Appendixes

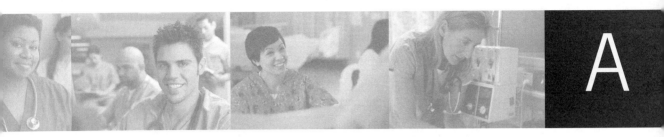

Project Management Guide

Appendix A: Project Management Guide

Initial EBP Question:
EBP Team Leader(s):
EBP Team Members:

Activities	Start Date	Days Required	End Date	Person Assigned	Milestone	Comment / Resources Required
PRACTICE QUESTION:						
Step 1: Recruit interprofessional team						
Step 2: Develop and refine the EBP question						
Step 3: Define the scope of the EBP question and identify stakeholders						
Step 4: Determine responsibility for project leadership						
Step 5: Schedule team meetings						
EVIDENCE:						
Step 6: Conduct internal and external search for evidence						
Step 7: Appraise the level and quality of each piece of evidence						
Step 8: Summarize the individual evidence						
Step 9: Synthesize overall strength and quality of evidence						
Step 10: Develop recommendations for change based on evidence synthesis □ Strong, compelling evidence, consistent results □ Good evidence, consistent results □ Good evidence, conflicting results □ Insufficient or absent evidence						
TRANSLATION:						
Step 11: Determine fit, feasibility, and appropriateness of recommendation(s) for translation path						
Step 12: Create action plan						
Step 13: Secure support and resources to implement action plan						
Step 14: Implement action plan						
Step 15: Evaluate outcomes						
Step 16: Report outcomes to stakeholders						
Step 17: Identify next steps						
Step 18: Disseminate findings						

© The Johns Hopkins Hospital/The Johns Hopkins University

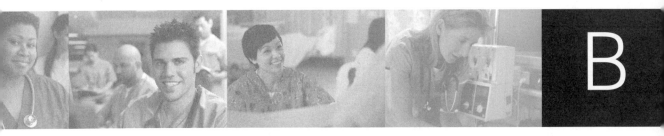

Question Development Tool

Appendix B: Question Development Tool

1. What is the problem and why is it important?

2. What is the current practice?

3. What is the focus of the problem?

☐ Clinical   ☐ Educational   ☐ Administrative

4. How was the problem identified?   (Check all that apply)

☐ Safety/risk management concerns
☐ Quality concerns (efficiency, effectiveness, timeliness, equity, patient-centeredness)
☐ Unsatisfactory patient, staff, or organizational outcomes
☐ Variations in practice within the setting

☐ Variations in practice compared with external organizations
☐ Evidence validation for current practice
☐ Financial concerns

5. What is the scope of the problem?

☐ Individual   ☐ Population   ☐ Institution/system

6. What are the PICO components?

P – (Patient, population, problem):

I – (Intervention):

C – (Comparison with other interventions, if applicable):

O – (Outcomes that include metrics for evaluating results):

7. Initial EBP question:

8. List possible search terms, databases to search, and search strategies:

9. What evidence must be gathered?   (Check all that apply)

☐ Literature search
☐ Standards (regulatory, professional, community)
☐ Guidelines
☐ Expert opinion

☐ Patient/family preferences
☐ Clinical expertise
☐ Organizational data

© The Johns Hopkins Hospital/The Johns Hopkins University

Directions for Use of the Question Development Tool

Purpose: This form is used to develop an answerable question and to guide the team in the evidence search process. The question, search terms and strategy, and sources of evidence can be revised as the EBP team refines the EBP project focus.

What is the problem and why is it important? Indicate why the project was undertaken. What led the team to seek evidence? Make sure the problem statement defines the actual problem and does not include a solution statement.

What is the current practice? Define the current practice as it relates to the problem.

What is the focus of the problem? Is the problem a clinical concern (e.g., preventing blood stream infections); an educational concern (e.g., discharge teaching for patients); or an administrative concern (e.g., safety of 12-hour nursing shifts)?

How was the problem identified? Check the statements that describe how the problem was identified.

What is the scope of the problem? Does the problem look at an individual (e.g., clinician, patient, family member); a population (e.g., adult cardiac patients, recovery room nurses); or an institution/system (e.g., patient transportation, patient or staff satisfaction)?

What are the PICO components?

- **P** (patient, population, problem) e.g., age, sex, setting, ethnicity, condition, disease, type of patient, or population

- **I** (intervention) e.g., treatment, medications, education, diagnostic tests or best practice(s)

- **C** (comparison with other interventions or current practice) may not be applicable if your question is looking for best practice.

- **O** (outcome) stated in measurable terms, expected outcomes based on the intervention identified, e.g., decrease in fall rate, decrease in length of stay, increase in patient satisfaction.

Initial EBP Question. A starting question that can be refined and adjusted as the team searches through the literature.

List possible search terms. Using PICO components and the initial EBP question, list relevant terms to begin the evidence search. Terms can be added or adjusted as the evidence search continues. Document the search terms, strategy, and databases searched in sufficient detail for replication.

What evidence must be gathered? Check the types of evidence the team will gather based on the PICO and initial EBP question.

© The Johns Hopkins Hospital/The Johns Hopkins University

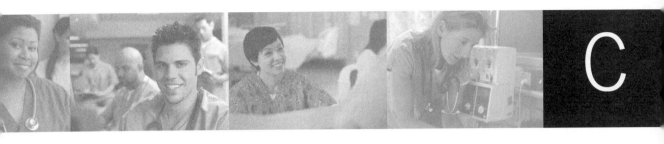

Evidence Level and
Quality Guide

Appendix C: Evidence Level and Quality Guide

Evidence Levels	Quality Guides
Level I Experimental study, randomized controlled trial (RCT) Systematic review of RCTs, with or without meta-analysis	**A High quality:** Consistent, generalizable results; sufficient sample size for the study design; adequate control; definitive conclusions; consistent recommendations based on comprehensive literature review that includes thorough reference to scientific evidence **B Good quality:** Reasonably consistent results; sufficient sample size for the study design; some control, fairly definitive conclusions; reasonably consistent recommendations based on fairly comprehensive literature review that includes some reference to scientific evidence **C Low quality or major flaws:** Little evidence with inconsistent results; insufficient sample size for the study design; conclusions cannot be drawn
Level II Quasi-experimental study Systematic review of a combination of RCTs and quasi-experimental, or quasi-experimental studies only, with or without meta-analysis	
Level III Non-experimental study Systematic review of a combination of RCTs, quasi-experimental and non-experimental studies, or non-experimental studies only, with or without meta-analysis Qualitative study or systematic review with or without a meta-synthesis	
Level IV Opinion of respected authorities and/or nationally recognized expert committees/consensus panels based on scientific evidence Includes: • Clinical practice guidelines • Consensus panels	**A High quality:** Material officially sponsored by a professional, public, private organization, or government agency; documentation of a systematic literature search strategy; consistent results with sufficient numbers of well-designed studies; criteria-based evaluation of overall scientific strength and quality of included studies and definitive conclusions; national expertise is clearly evident; developed or revised within the last 5 years **B Good quality:** Material officially sponsored by a professional, public, private organization, or government agency; reasonably thorough and appropriate systematic literature search strategy; reasonably consistent results, sufficient numbers of well-designed studies; evaluation of strengths and limitations of included studies with fairly definitive conclusions; national expertise is clearly evident; developed or revised within the last 5 years **C Low quality or major flaws:** Material not sponsored by an official organization or agency; undefined, poorly defined, or limited literature search strategy; no evaluation of strengths and limitations of included studies, insufficient evidence with inconsistent results, conclusions cannot be drawn; not revised within the last 5 years

© The Johns Hopkins Hospital/The Johns Hopkins University

Appendix C: Evidence Level and Quality Guide

Level V

Based on experiential and non-research evidence

Includes:

- Literature reviews
- Quality improvement, program or financial evaluation
- Case reports
- Opinion of nationally recognized experts(s) based on experiential evidence

Organizational Experience:

A **High quality:** Clear aims and objectives; consistent results across multiple settings; formal quality improvement, financial or program evaluation methods used; definitive conclusions; consistent recommendations with thorough reference to scientific evidence

B **Good quality:** Clear aims and objectives; consistent results in a single setting; formal quality improvement or financial or program evaluation methods used; reasonably consistent recommendations with some reference to scientific evidence

C **Low quality or major flaws:** Unclear or missing aims and objectives; inconsistent results; poorly defined quality improvement, financial or program evaluation methods; recommendations cannot be made

Literature Review, Expert Opinion, Case Report, Community Standard, Clinician Experience, Consumer Preference:

A **High quality:** Expertise is clearly evident; draws definitive conclusions; provides scientific rationale; thought leader(s) in the field

B **Good quality:** Expertise appears to be credible; draws fairly definitive conclusions; provides logical argument for opinions

C **Low quality or major flaws:** Expertise is not discernable or is dubious; conclusions cannot be drawn

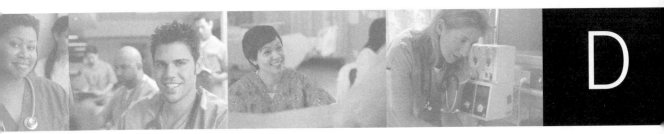

Practice Question, Evidence, and Translation Process (PET)

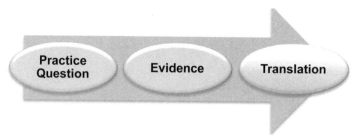

PRACTICE QUESTION

Step 1: Recruit interprofessional team
Step 2: Develop and refine the EBP question
Step 3: Define the scope of the EBP question and identify stakeholders
Step 4: Determine responsibility for project leadership
Step 5: Schedule team meetings

EVIDENCE

Step 6: Conduct internal and external search for evidence
Step 7: Appraise the level and quality of each piece of evidence
Step 8: Summarize the individual evidence
Step 9: Synthesize overall strength and quality of evidence
Step 10: Develop recommendations for change based on evidence synthesis
- Strong, compelling evidence, consistent results
- Good evidence, consistent results
- Good evidence, conflicting results
- Insufficient or absent evidence

TRANSLATION

Step 11: Determine fit, feasibility, and appropriateness of recommendation(s)
        for translation path
Step 12: Create action plan
Step 13: Secure support and resources to implement action plan
Step 14: Implement action plan
Step 15: Evaluate outcomes
Step 16: Report outcomes to stakeholders
Step 17: Identify next steps
Step 18: Disseminate findings

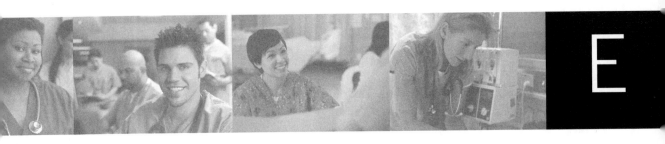

Research Evidence
Appraisal Tool

Appendix E: Research Evidence Appraisal Tool

Evidence Level and Quality:_____

Article Title:	Number:
Author(s):	Publication Date:
Journal:	

Setting:	Sample (Composition & size):

Does this evidence address my EBP question?	☐Yes	☐No Do not proceed with appraisal of this evidence

Level of Evidence (Study Design)

A. Is this a report of a single research study? **If No, go to B.**	☐Yes	☐No
1. Was there an intervention?	☐Yes	☐No
2. Was there a control group?	☐Yes	☐No
3. Were study participants randomly assigned to the intervention and control groups?	☐Yes	☐No

If Yes to all three, this is a Randomized Controlled Trial (RCT) or Experimental Study   → ☐ LEVEL I

If Yes to #1 and #2 and No to #3, OR Yes to #1 and No to #2 and #3, this is Quasi Experimental (some degree of investigator control, some manipulation of an independent variable, lacks random assignment to groups, may have a control group)   → ☐ LEVEL II

If No to #1, #2, and #3, this is Non-Experimental (no manipulation of independent variable, can be descriptive, comparative, or correlational, often uses secondary data) **or Qualitative** (exploratory in nature such as interviews or focus groups, a starting point for studies for which little research currently exists, has small sample sizes, may use results to design empirical studies)   → ☐ LEVEL III

NEXT, COMPLETE THE BOTTOM SECTION ON THE FOLLOWING PAGE, "STUDY FINDINGS THAT HELP YOU ANSWER THE EBP QUESTION"

© The Johns Hopkins Hospital/The Johns Hopkins University

Appendix E: Research Evidence Appraisal Tool

B. Is this a summary of multiple research studies? *If No, go to Non-Research Evidence Appraisal Form.*	☐Yes	☐No
1. Does it employ a comprehensive search strategy and rigorous appraisal method (**Systematic Review**)? *If No, use Non-Research Evidence Appraisal Tool; if Yes:*	☐Yes	☐No
a. Does it combine and analyze results from the studies to generate a new statistic (effect size)? (**Systematic review with meta-analysis**)	☐Yes	☐No
b. Does it analyze and synthesize concepts from qualitative studies? (**Systematic review with meta-synthesis**)	☐Yes	☐No

      If Yes to either a or b, go to #2B below.

  2. For Systematic Reviews and Systematic Reviews with meta-analysis or meta-synthesis:

      a. Are all studies included RCTs?   ➔ ☐ LEVEL I

      b. Are the studies a combination of RCTs and quasi-experimental or quasi-experimental only?   ➔ ☐ LEVEL II

      c. Are the studies a combination of RCTs, quasi-experimental and non-experimental or non-experimental only?   ➔ ☐ LEVEL III

      d. Are any or all of the included studies qualitative?   ➔ ☐ LEVEL III

COMPLETE THE NEXT SECTION, "STUDY FINDINGS THAT HELP YOU ANSWER THE EBP QUESTION"

STUDY FINDINGS THAT HELP YOU ANSWER THE EBP QUESTION:

NOW COMPLETE THE FOLLOWING PAGE, "QUALITY APPRAISAL OF RESEARCH STUDIES", AND ASSIGN A QUALITY SCORE TO YOUR ARTICLE

© The Johns Hopkins Hospital/The Johns Hopkins University

Appendix E: Research Evidence Appraisal Tool

Quality Appraisal of Research Studies			
• Does the researcher identify what is known and not known about the problem and how the study will address any gaps in knowledge?	☐Yes	☐No	
• Was the purpose of the study clearly presented?	☐Yes	☐No	
• Was the literature review current (most sources within last 5 years or classic)?	☐Yes	☐No	
• Was sample size sufficient based on study design and rationale?	☐Yes	☐No	
• If there is a control group:			
○ Were the characteristics and/or demographics similar in both the control and intervention groups?	☐Yes	☐No	☐NA
○ If multiple settings were used, were the settings similar?	☐Yes	☐No	☐NA
○ Were all groups equally treated except for the intervention group(s)?	☐Yes	☐No	☐NA
• Are data collection methods described clearly?	☐Yes	☐No	
• Were the instruments reliable (Cronbach's α [alpha] ≥ 0.70)?	☐Yes	☐No	☐NA
• Was instrument validity discussed?	☐Yes	☐No	☐NA
• If surveys/questionnaires were used, was the response rate ≥ 25%?	☐Yes	☐No	☐NA
• Were the results presented clearly?	☐Yes	☐No	
• If tables were presented, was the narrative consistent with the table content?	☐Yes	☐No	☐NA
• Were study limitations identified and addressed?	☐Yes	☐No	
• Were conclusions based on results?	☐Yes	☐No	

Quality Appraisal of Systematic Review with or without Meta-Analysis or Meta-Synthesis		
• Was the purpose of the systematic review clearly stated?	☐Yes	☐No
• Were reports comprehensive, with reproducible search strategy?	☐Yes	☐No
○ Key search terms stated	☐Yes	☐No
○ Multiple databases searched and identified	☐Yes	☐No
○ Inclusion and exclusion criteria stated	☐Yes	☐No
• Was there a flow diagram showing the number of studies eliminated at each level of review?	☐Yes	☐No
• Were details of included studies presented (design, sample, methods, results, outcomes, strengths and limitations)?	☐Yes	☐No
• Were methods for appraising the strength of evidence (level and quality) described?	☐Yes	☐No
• Were conclusions based on results?	☐Yes	☐No
○ Results were interpreted	☐Yes	☐No
○ Conclusions flowed logically from the interpretation and systematic review question	☐Yes	☐No
• Did the systematic review include both a section addressing limitations and how they were addressed?	☐Yes	☐No

QUALITY RATING BASED ON QUALITY APPRAISAL

A **High quality:** consistent, generalizable results; sufficient sample size for the study design; adequate control; definitive conclusions; consistent recommendations based on comprehensive literature review that includes thorough reference to scientific evidence

B **Good quality:** reasonably consistent results; sufficient sample size for the study design; some control, and fairly definitive conclusions; reasonably consistent recommendations based on fairly comprehensive literature review that includes some reference to scientific evidence

C **Low quality or major flaws:** little evidence with inconsistent results; insufficient sample size for the study design; conclusions cannot be drawn

© The Johns Hopkins Hospital/The Johns Hopkins University

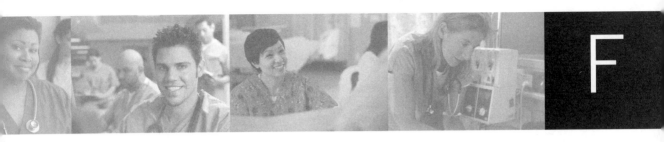

Non-Research Evidence
Appraisal Tool

Appendix F: Non-Research Evidence Appraisal Tool

Evidence Level & Quality:_____

Article Title:	Number:
Author(s):	Publication Date:
Journal:	

Does this evidence address the EBP question?	☐Yes	☐No Do not proceed with appraisal of this evidence

☐ **Clinical Practice Guidelines:** Systematically developed recommendations from nationally recognized experts based on research evidence or expert consensus panel. **LEVEL IV**

☐ **Consensus or Position Statement:** Systematically developed recommendations based on research and nationally recognized expert opinion that guides members of a professional organization in decision-making for an issue of concern. **LEVEL IV**

• Are the types of evidence included identified?	☐Yes	☐No
• Were appropriate stakeholders involved in the development of recommendations?	☐Yes	☐No
• Are groups to which recommendations apply and do not apply clearly stated?	☐Yes	☐No
• Have potential biases been eliminated?	☐Yes	☐No
• Were recommendations valid (reproducible search, expert consensus, independent review, current, and level of supporting evidence identified for each recommendation)?	☐Yes	☐No
• Were the recommendations supported by evidence?	☐Yes	☐No
• Are recommendations clear?	☐Yes	☐No

☐ **Literature Review:** Summary of published literature without systematic appraisal of evidence quality or strength. **LEVEL V**

• Is subject matter to be reviewed clearly stated?	☐Yes	☐No
• Is relevant, up-to-date literature included in the review (most sources within last 5 years or classic)?	☐Yes	☐No
• Is there a meaningful analysis of the conclusions in the literature?	☐Yes	☐No
• Are gaps in the literature identified?	☐Yes	☐No
• Are recommendations made for future practice or study?	☐Yes	☐No

☐ **Expert Opinion:** Opinion of one or more individuals based on clinical expertise. **LEVEL V**

• Has the individual published or presented on the topic?	☐Yes	☐No
• Is author's opinion based on scientific evidence?	☐Yes	☐No
• Is the author's opinion clearly stated?	☐Yes	☐No
• Are potential biases acknowledged?	☐Yes	☐No

Appendix F: Non-Research Evidence Appraisal Tool

Organizational Experience:			
☐ **Quality Improvement:** Cyclical method to examine organization-specific processes at the local level. **LEVEL V**			
☐ **Financial Evaluation:** Economic evaluation that applies analytic techniques to identify, measure, and compare the cost and outcomes of two or more alternative programs or interventions. **LEVEL V**			
☐ **Program Evaluation:** Systematic assessment of the processes and/or outcomes of a program and can involve both quantitative and qualitative methods. **LEVEL V**			

Setting:	Sample (composition/size):		
• Was the aim of the project clearly stated?		☐Yes	☐No
• Was the method adequately described?		☐Yes	☐No
• Were process or outcome measures identified?		☐Yes	☐No
• Were results adequately described?		☐Yes	☐No
• Was interpretation clear and appropriate?		☐Yes	☐No
• Are components of cost/benefit analysis described?		☐Yes	☐No ☐N/A

☐ **Case Report:** In-depth look at a person, group, or other social unit. **LEVEL V**		
• Is the purpose of the case report clearly stated?	☐Yes	☐No
• Is the case report clearly presented?	☐Yes	☐No
• Are the findings of the case report supported by relevant theory or research?	☐Yes	☐No
• Are the recommendations clearly stated and linked to the findings?	☐Yes	☐No

Community Standard, Clinician Experience, or Consumer Preference			
☐ **Community Standard:** Current practice for comparable settings in the community **LEVEL V**			
☐ **Clinician Experience:** Knowledge gained through practice experience **LEVEL V**			
☐ **Consumer Preference:** Knowledge gained through life experience **LEVEL V**			

Information Source(s):	Number of Sources:		
• Source of information has credible experience.		☐Yes	☐No
• Opinions are clearly stated.		☐Yes	☐No ☐N/A
• Identified practices are consistent.		☐Yes	☐No ☐N/A

Findings that help you answer the EBP question:

Appendix F: Non-Research Evidence Appraisal Tool

QUALITY RATING FOR CLINICAL PRACTICE GUIDELINES, CONSENSUS OR POSITION STATEMENTS (LEVEL IV)

A <u>High quality:</u> Material officially sponsored by a professional, public, private organization, or government agency; documentation of a systematic literature search strategy; consistent results with sufficient numbers of well-designed studies; criteria-based evaluation of overall scientific strength and quality of included studies and definitive conclusions; national expertise is clearly evident; developed or revised within the last 5 years.

B <u>Good quality:</u> Material officially sponsored by a professional, public, private organization, or government agency; reasonably thorough and appropriate systematic literature search strategy; reasonably consistent results, sufficient numbers of well-designed studies; evaluation of strengths and limitations of included studies with fairly definitive conclusions; national expertise is clearly evident; developed or revised within the last 5 years.

C <u>Low quality or major flaws:</u> Material not sponsored by an official organization or agency; undefined, poorly defined, or limited literature search strategy; no evaluation of strengths and limitations of included studies, insufficient evidence with inconsistent results, conclusions cannot be drawn; not revised within the last 5 years.

QUALITY RATING FOR ORGANIZATIONAL EXPERIENCE (LEVEL V)

A <u>High quality:</u> Clear aims and objectives; consistent results across multiple settings; formal quality improvement or financial evaluation methods used; definitive conclusions; consistent recommendations with thorough reference to scientific evidence

B <u>Good quality:</u> Clear aims and objectives; formal quality improvement or financial evaluation methods used; consistent results in a single setting; reasonably consistent recommendations with some reference to scientific evidence

C <u>Low quality or major flaws:</u> Unclear or missing aims and objectives; inconsistent results; poorly defined quality improvement/financial analysis method; recommendations cannot be made

---

QUALITY RATING FOR LITERATURE REVIEW, EXPERT OPINION, COMMUNITY STANDARD, CLINICIAN EXPERIENCE, CONSUMER PREFERENCE (LEVEL V)

A <u>High quality:</u> Expertise is clearly evident; draws definitive conclusions; provides scientific rationale; thought leader in the field

B <u>Good quality:</u> Expertise appears to be credible; draws fairly definitive conclusions; provides logical argument for opinions

C <u>Low quality or major flaws:</u> Expertise is not discernable or is dubious; conclusions cannot be drawn

---

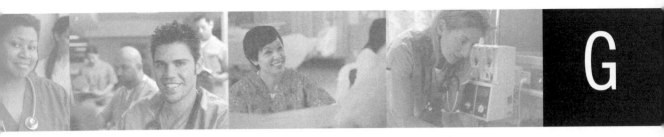

Individual Evidence Summary Tool

Appendix G: Individual Evidence Summary Tool

EBP Question:

Date:

Article #	Author & Date	Evidence Type	Sample, Sample Size & Setting	Study findings that help answer the EBP question	Limitations	Evidence Level & Quality
			☐ N/A			
			☐ N/A			
			☐ N/A			
			☐ N/A			
			☐ N/A			
			☐ N/A			
			☐ N/A			
			☐ N/A			
			☐ N/A			

Attach a reference list with full citations of articles reviewed for this EBP question.

© The Johns Hopkins Hospital/The Johns Hopkins University

Appendix G: Individual Evidence Summary Tool

Directions for Use of the Individual Evidence Summary Tool

Purpose: This form is used to document the results of evidence appraisal in preparation for evidence synthesis. It provides the EBP team with documentation of the sources of evidence used, the year the evidence was published or otherwise communicated, the information gathered from each evidence source that helps the team answer the EBP question, and the level and quality of each source of evidence.

Header: Record the EBP question and date of the EBP project for reference.

Article #: Assign a number to each reviewed source of evidence. This organizes the Individual Evidence Summary and provides an easy way to reference articles.

Author and Date: Indicate the last name of first author, or the evidence source and the publication/communication date. It is important to list both author/evidence source and date because several documents may be from the same source.

Evidence Type: Indicate the type of evidence reviewed (*example: RCT, meta-analysis, qualitative, systematic review, case study, narrative literature review*).

Sample, Sample Size, and Setting: This is only applicable for evidence levels I, II, III, and level V quality improvement, financial or program evaluation. Provides a quick view of the population, number of participants, and where the study took place.

Study findings that help answer the EBP question: Although there may be many points of interest to the reviewer, list only findings that directly apply to the EBP question.

Limitations: Include information that may or may not be within the text of the article regarding drawbacks of the piece of evidence. The evidence may list limitations, or it may be evident to you as you review the evidence that an important point is missed, or the sample does not apply to the population of interest.

Evidence Level and Quality: Using information from the individual appraisal tools, transfer the evidence level and quality rating into this column.

© The Johns Hopkins Hospital/The Johns Hopkins University

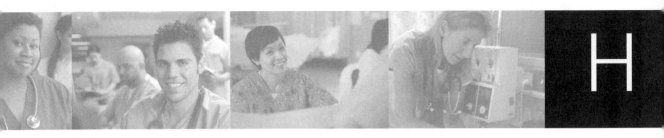

Synthesis and Recommendations Tool

Appendix H: Synthesis and Recommendations Tool

EBP Question:

Date:

Category (Level Type)	Total Number of Sources/Level	Overall Quality Rating	Synthesis of Findings Evidence That Answers the EBP Question
Level I · Experimental study · Randomized Controlled Trial (RCT) · Systematic review of RCTs with or without meta-analysis			
Level II · Quasi-experimental studies · Systematic review of a combination of RCTs and quasi-experimental studies, or quasi-experimental studies only, with or without meta-analysis			
Level III · Non-experimental study · Systematic review of a combination of RCTs, quasi-experimental, and non-experimental studies, or non-experimental studies only, with or without meta-analysis · Qualitative study or systematic review of qualitative studies with or without meta-synthesis			
Level IV · Opinion of respected authorities and/or reports of nationally recognized expert committees/consensus panels based on scientific evidence			
Level V · Evidence obtained from literature reviews, quality improvement, program evaluation, financial evaluation, or case reports · Opinion of nationally recognized expert(s) based on experiential evidence			

© The Johns Hopkins Hospital/The Johns Hopkins University

Appendix H: Synthesis and Recommendations Tool

EBP Question:

Date:

Recommendations Based on Evidence Synthesis and Selected Translation Pathway

Directions for Use of This Form

Purpose: This form is used to compile the results of the evidence appraisal to answer the EBP question. The pertinent findings for each level of evidence are synthesized, and a quality rating is assigned to each level.

Total Number of Sources per Level: Record the number of sources of evidence for each level.

Overall Quality Rating: Summarize the overall quality of evidence for each level. Use the "Evidence Level and Quality Guide" (Appendix C) to rate the quality of evidence.

Synthesis of Findings: Evidence That Answers the EBP Question

- Include only findings from evidence of A or B quality.
- Include only statements that directly answer the EBP question.
- Summarize findings within each level of evidence.
- Record article number(s) from individual evidence summary in parentheses next to each statement so it is easy to identify the source of the finding.

Develop Recommendations Based on Evidence Synthesis and the Selected Translation Pathway: Review the synthesis of findings and determine which of the following four pathways to translation represents the overall strength of the evidence:

- Strong, compelling evidence, consistent results: solid indication for a practice change.
- Good and consistent evidence: consider pilot of change or further investigation.
- Good but conflicting evidence: no indication for practice change; consider further investigation for new evidence or develop a research study.
- Little or no evidence: no indication for practice change; consider further investigation for new evidence or develop a research study or discontinue project.

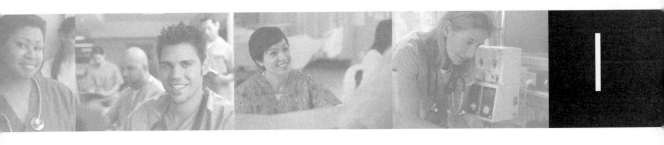

Synthesis of Evidence Guide

Appendix I: Synthesis of Evidence Guide

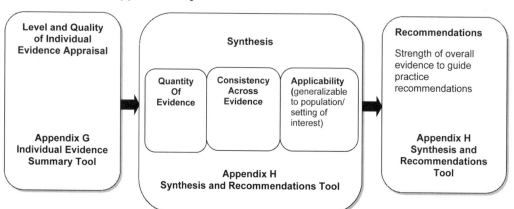

Key Points:

- Synthesis of evidence begins with reviewing and reflecting on the quality appraisal of the individual pieces of evidence for each level (I-V). Reflection involves looking at the meaning and relevance of the evidence.
    - What meaning and relevance does the evidence have for the question?
    - Does the evidence help to answer the question?
    - Does the evidence enhance the team's knowledge?

- The same criteria used to synthesize individual evidence can also be used for synthesizing the overall quality of evidence (see Appendix C, Evidence Level and Quality Guide).

- Synthesis involves summarizing the quantity of evidence for each level. The assessment of quantity is important because multiple pieces of level I and II evidence, with consistent findings, allow the EBP team to have greater confidence in recommending a practice change.
    - Evidence synthesis is best done through group discussion; team members share their different perspectives and use critical thinking to arrive at a judgment based on consensus.
    - This process involves both subjective and objective reflection and reasoning.

- EBP teams often find that level I evidence is not available to answer their practice questions. The team should proceed cautiously in making practice changes based on level II and III evidence. For these levels, recommendation(s) typically include doing a pilot to test the recommendation(s) before deciding to implement a full scale change.

- Generally, practice changes are not made on level V evidence alone. However, teams have a variety of options for actions that include, but are not limited to: awareness campaigns, conducting informational and educational updates, monitoring evidence sources for new information, or designing a research study.

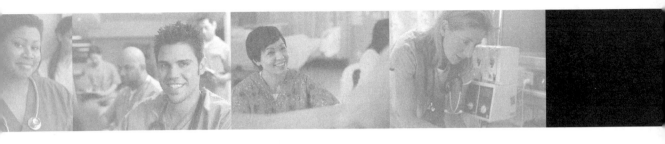

Index

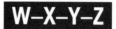

W–X–Y–Z

U–V